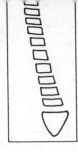

Contents

Back Pain

A handbook for sufferers

Back Pain

A handbook for sufferers

Loïc Burn & John Paterson

Foreword by Ian Haslock

Headway · Hodder & Stoughton

The authors and publishers would like to thank Jennifer Brown for her anatomical drawings, *The Independent on Sunday* for permission to reproduce the article on page 50 and Christina Jansen and Antonio Moreno for the cover photograph.

British Library Cataloguing in Publication Data

Burn, Loïc
   Back Pain: A Handbook for Sufferers
   I. Title   II. Paterson, John K.
   616.73

   ISBN 0-340-59762-3

First published 1993
Impression number 10 9 8 7 6 5 4 3 2 1
Year 1988 1997 1996 1995 1994 1993

© 1993 Loïc Burn & John Paterson

Typeset by Rowland Phototypesetting Limited, Bury St Edmunds, Suffolk. Printed in Great Britain for the educational publishing division of Hodder & Stoughton Limited, Mill Road, Dunton Green, Sevenoaks, Kent TN13 2YA by Cox and Wyman Limited.

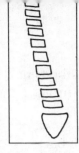

Foreword

Back pain is one of the commonest symptoms we suffer. Almost everyone has pain in their back at some time, but most episodes settle with little or no treatment. Those who need treatment suffer from a number of frustrations. Conventional medical treatment is unsuccessful in some people, and they are then presented with a vast range of alternative practitioners, all of whom claim to have the answer to their problem. Well-meaning friends and acquaintances add their own advice, a lot of which is contradictory, with the result that the back pain sufferer becomes totally confused regarding the right path to take.

Most doctors now accept the benefits of patients knowing as much as possible about their own disease. Many hospital physiotherapy departments use self-knowledge as an important part of their 'Back School' approach to back pain management. Unfortunately, many books on back pain fail to inform the reader objectively, but simply express the authors' prejudices as facts; theories for which there is no evidence may be presented as if they were scientifically proved, and treatments whose effects have never been exposed to proper assessment are presented as of proved effectiveness. Most worrying is the tendency of many such books to blame the sufferer who fails to respond to the 'curative' treatment rather than admit that no one universal remedy for back pain exists.

This book is a refreshing change. Its authors are experienced general practitioners who practise and teach manipulative methods of treatment. They are open about their own prejudices and working methods, and assess them as objectively as they assess the methods of others. Their language is clear and their guide through the maze of conventional medical and alternative methods of treatment is illuminated by a useful glossary of the terms which confuse so many people with back pain. Readers of this book will understand their backs better and will have a greater knowledge of the ways in which they can help themselves to overcome their problems. They will also be able to choose in a more discriminating way among the many forms of treatment on offer, and use the knowledge they have gained to make the best use of every consultation and each form of treatment they are given.

Ian Haslock
Consultant Rheumatologist, South Tees District.
Past President, British Society for Rheumatology.

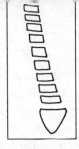

Introduction

This book is for people who suffer from back pain but is also a sequel to a text we have recently published for the medical profession called *Musculoskeletal Medicine – The Spine*. We feel that the scale of the back pain problem is so great that books are necessary both for doctors and patients. Doctors, world-wide, receive little training in back pain diagnosis and management and it is acknowledged by all medical authorities that this sad situation has to be corrected. Lack of appropriate training means that your family doctor may not be well informed about back pain. If you went to your doctor with chronic bronchitis or heart disease, you would expect them to be knowledgeable and able to give you detailed and helpful advice. With your back pain, this is unlikely.

Because back pain is largely misunderstood, there is another, almost bizarre, characteristic in this field. In no other area of medicine are there so many different ideas, vocabularies, jargons, cults and groups of people contending to treat you as there are in back pain. You will have heard of 'osteopaths', but who has ever heard of a 'cardiopath' to treat your heart complaint or a 'diabetopath' to deal with your diabetes? The many types of clinician may leave you in something of a quandary. So this book provides you with a guide to all these people, their beliefs and treatments and suggests who to go to for safe advice. Above all, we suggest who and what to avoid!

We also explain the confusing terms used to describe your back, in order to guide you through what is known about its structure.

We also give you up-to-date psychological information, so that you may form a realistic and objective picture of the mental aspects of back pain.

In short, we present a review of the current state of play with regard to back pain. Our main reason for doing this is that ignorance causes confusion, misunderstanding, anxiety and a sense of helplessness. If you have a mistaken picture, or no idea at all, as to what is going on with your back, this must make an already difficult situation worse for you.

Finally we discuss the *chronic pain state*. This state is now recognised by doctors, world-wide. If you have the bad luck to have chronic or frequently recurring attacks of back pain, how can you cope? We give advice, but how you cope depends upon how *you* act upon this advice.

We are very grateful for the suggestions that many colleagues and former patients have made. We are also indebted to Kluwer Academic Publishers, for allowing us to draw upon books we have written for the medical profession, and to Dr Mervyn Bryn-Jones, Executive Director of the National Back Pain Association, for writing a section describing the activities of that organisation.

Finally we owe a great debt of gratitude to Dr Ian Haslock, past president of the British Society for Rheumatology, for doing us the honour of writing a foreword to this book.

Loïc Burn
John Paterson   London, 26th March, 1993

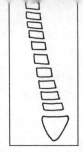

CHAPTER I

Scale of the problem

SCOPE OF THE PROBLEM IN THE NATIONAL ECONOMY

Before the age of 55, approximately 8 out of 10 people suffer back pain so severe that they are forced to see a doctor, so none will deny that back pain is a major social problem. Every day some 90,000 people register as sick and stay away from work as a result of back pain and · this figure has been growing steadily over the past few years. According to figures from the National Back Pain Association, 1992, the cost each year in lost production, sickness benefits and medical treatment is running at about £3000 million and is set to increase.

The available figures come from different sources, and they are not always exactly the same, but they do rub in the fact that the problem is enormous and still growing. The cost of sickness or accident benefit and medical treatment, whether private or within the NHS, is met by you, either straight from your pocket, through an insurance policy or as a part of your tax burden. Back pain is a huge cost to the whole economy – industry, business and individuals.

The number of days at work lost due to back pain doubled from 15 to 30 million between 1970 and 1980, and again from 30 to 60 million by 1990. In 1991 the number of working days lost to back pain was 67 million. This ticking time bomb is a major reason for back pain having been identified in the White Paper *The Health of the Nation, July 1992* as a key area for concern. The Government has now entered into discussions with interested bodies on how to tackle the problem, and a concerted effort to educate people about their backs can be expected.

SCOPE OF THE PROBLEM FOR DOCTORS

Back pain is a huge problem for the economy and it is also a huge problem for the medical profession. A number of features make back pain especially difficult for doctors:

- There are very many causes of back pain and this makes diagnosis extremely difficult. The causes of back pain are reviewed in chapter 2. We examine diagnosis in chapter 6.
- Your GP is likely to have received inadequate training about back pain, so he or she may well lack confidence when treating you. Do not blame your GP if he or she seems uncertain; the whole medical establishment is at fault for not ensuring adequate training for students and post-graduate training for GPs.
- Back pain is unlike any other branch of medicine because in this field your doctor is competing with a range of alternative and complementary practitioners. The fact that so many people claim to know all about back pain is confusing for your doctor, as well as for you. We review the people who may help you in chapter 9.
- Like you, doctors badly need reliable information about back pain problems, based on what is at present *known* to be true. This book aims to supply reliable information which will be of use to everybody.

SCOPE OF THE PROBLEM FOR YOU

We have seen that back pain is a huge problem for the economy and for doctors. Of course, if you suffer from it, back pain is also a huge problem for you, presenting challenges which affect every aspect of your life, perhaps making you feel angry and resentful, as this account from a middle-aged, professional man makes clear.

A sufferer speaks out

I have had back pain on and off for ten years. I usually get it once or twice a year and it mostly clears up in 48 hours or, at any rate, in less than a week. Sometimes it lasts far longer and is so severe that I can't work. One attack lasted more than six weeks. I was very disappointed in my GP. He never examined me and only asked where the pain was and whether I had done anything to bring it on. He gave me two different sorts of pain-killer and, while neither helped, one gave me indigestion. He told me to stay in bed but that didn't help either. Finally he had an X-ray taken and said that it showed a lot of wear and tear and that I would have to learn to put up with it. I didn't find that very helpful, and it didn't even make much sense as most of the time I am pain-free. After all, if it was 'wear and tear' you would have thought that it would be there all the time, and it isn't.

I asked my friends what I should do and got a lot of conflicting advice. In the end I went to an osteopath and he helped me. But the next bad attack that I got didn't respond to his treatment or to that of a chiropractor or an acupuncturist that I went to. It finally cleared up on its own. They all told me that my pain was due to different causes and this I found very confusing and unsatisfactory, although sometimes their treatments helped.

I dread another severe attack because I don't know how

long it will last, and although my colleagues are understanding I am worried about the effects on my working life.

I wonder whether my family think I'm putting it on. I even wonder sometimes if I am imagining it.

I feel so helpless in all this as nobody seems to know what is wrong and people give me completely different explanations. One so-called clinician told me that I had six different discs and that he was going to put them back, one every treatment sessions.

I am not in pain now, but how long will I be pain-free and what do I do if I get another bad attack?

This account touches on some of the problems we will discuss in this book – sufferers' relationships with their doctors, the range of advice on offer, effects of back pain on a sufferer's career, family and mental health.

The difficulties may seem awesome, but never forget that there are organisations which may help you – organisations such as *Arthritis Care* and the *National Back Pain Association*. We give the addresses of organisations which may help you in appendix 5. You have people you can turn to when you need help, but most of all you may want to help yourself. Helping yourself to understand your problem and to lessen its hold over your life is what this book is all about.

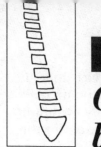

CHAPTER 2

Causes of back pain

In this chapter we will look at some of the suspected causes of back pain – we say 'suspected' because it is very difficult to pin down causes in this area. We will examine two types of cause:

- General factors which may contribute to back pain.
- Suggested specific factors in cases of back pain.

GENERAL CONTRIBUTORY FACTORS

Work

Many possible causes of back pain have been suggested and carefully investigated. A number of general factors need to be taken into account such as your work. Physically heavy work, working in the same position for a long time, frequent bending and twisting, lifting and forceful movements, repetitive work, working in stooped positions and work with vibration all increase the load on your spine. But of course more than one working 'style' may be present at the same time, further confusing the situation.

Evolution

Even evolution has been suggested as a contributory cause of back pain, in particular mankind's habit of standing up and walking on two legs! But as we have been walking upright for about 4 million years, we really should have got used to it by now! It is worth noting that, in pre-historic times, man, the hunter–gatherer, undertook perhaps only 50 lifts a day, whereas since the industrial revolution workers have undertaken up to 5,000 lifts a day. Perhaps our socio—economic evolution towards a complex industrial society is a reason for the amount of back pain. These attractively simple theories for back pain have never been proved.

Age

Personal differences, for example age, are also thought to contribute to low back pain. Low back pain has been shown to be most frequent between the ages of 35 and 55. This is of great importance, because many doctors associate low back pain with degenerative spinal changes shown on X-ray in the elderly. In fact, after the age of 55, your chance of low back pain decreases.

Gender

Gender could also influence back pain, although the situation is confused. Disc surgery is twice as common in males as it is in females. Sickness absence is much more common in women doing heavy physical work than in men doing physical work. But disc surgery is happily rare, and relatively few women do heavy work. So conclusions about the role of gender in back pain are difficult to draw. The exception is back pain in pregnancy. We discuss this separately, in appendix 1.

Posture and fitness

Bad posture has often been put forward as a major cause of back pain, but surprisingly in no case has this been proved. However, what is clear is that posture is not static but continually changes, allowing the back and neck to move all the time. To stay in any one position may cause stiffness and pain. If you do some exercises regularly you are less likely to complain of back pain, but there is no evidence that muscle strength has a direct effect in back pain – many exceedingly fit people are sufferers.

SPECIFIC FACTORS

You might like to re-read this section when you have read chapters 3 and 4, where we deal with the structure of the back in some detail. The glossary explains the technical vocabulary we use throughout the book, some of it is introduced here.

The disc

There is a disc of cartilage between each of the bones, called the *vertebrae*, which make up your spine (see figure 1). The discs allow the vertebrae to move smoothly against each other, while also preventing them from wearing.

You will have heard of a *slipped disc* and may have heard of a *disc lesion*, a *disc protrusion* or a *prolapsed disc*. Disc lesion means only that there is something wrong with the disc – what precisely is wrong is not stated. Disc protrusion means that a part of the disc is sticking out from its proper place. A prolapsed disc is one which has been so badly damaged that part of it, the *nucleus pulposus*, has been squeezed out into the spinal canal (see figure 4). Here it may interfere with the nervous system, sometimes pressing on the spinal nerve cord or on a nerve root. Use of the term *slipped disc* causes much confusion. It came into use about 60 years ago, when an American surgeon discovered that he had removed part of a disc during an operation. He concluded that this must be the cause of lumbago and sciatica, an idea that was immediately taken up by doctors, world-wide, although it has never been proved that the disc is a common cause of back pain. More recent work has shown that the disc is at fault in no more than one case in twenty! It never slips!

The trapped nerve

A nerve from the spinal cord may become trapped between adjacent vertebrae. This is widely believed to be a common cause of back pain, though we now know that nerves can be trapped quite badly without causing any pain at all. So, if you have a trapped nerve, it may or may not cause you any pain. But we do know that most cases of back pain are NOT due to a trapped nerve.

Arthritis

Arthritis means inflammation of a joint and may result from injury, from infection, or from particular diseases, such as rheumatoid arthritis. Many forms of arthritis get completely better, with or without treatment, but to use the word to describe the changes we all experience in middle or later life is quite wrong. In fact, as already mentioned, we now know that, after the age of 55, backache becomes less common.

Other possible direct causes of back pain

Your pain can arise from a problem developing in one of many different structures, such as *ligaments, joint capsules, muscles* and *tendons*. Your doctor's problem is trying to tell which one is the source of the problem. Back pain can also be a symptom of stress-induced tension and of many minor infections and ailments, such as flu.

More serious problems may also lead to back pain. Shingles, kidney and gynaecological problems, as well as cancer affecting the vertebral bodies (often secondary to tumours elsewhere,) and tuberculosis of the spine can lead to back pain. These conditions are, happily, relatively rare, and can often be diagnosed quickly with the use of X-rays.

CONCLUSION

We have described some of the general factors influencing back pain and you can probably work out which of these apply in your case. We have also briefly described some of the most important specific causes of low back pain and you may have some idea that one of these is the source of your problem. However we emphasise that 9 out of 10 cases of back pain are what doctors call 'non-specific', in other words *no single cause can be found to explain them*. Much of this book is devoted to discussing what this means for you in the prevention, management and treatment of your non-specific back pain (for the rest of this book, when we say 'back pain' we mean 'non-specific back pain').

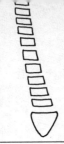

CHAPTER 3

How the back is built

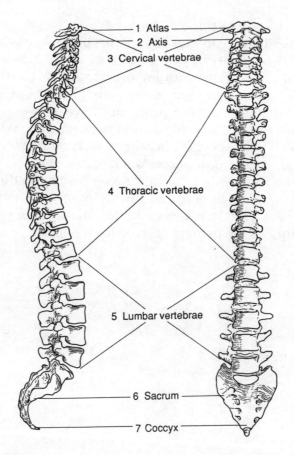

- 1 Atlas
- 2 Axis
- 3 Cervical vertebrae
- 4 Thoracic vertebrae
- 5 Lumbar vertebrae
- 6 Sacrum
- 7 Coccyx

figure 1

Between your skull and your pelvis there are 24 bones, the *vertebrae*. These are in 3 groups. There are 7 cervical (neck) vertebrae, 12 thoracic (middle back) vertebrae and 5 lumbar (lower back) vertebrae. This column 'stands' on your *sacrum*, which is made up of 5 fused vertebrae and is a triangular bone at the back of the pelvis, and the *coccyx* (a rudimentary tail made up of fused vertebrae at the base of the spine). This is shown in figure 1. The vertebrae that take the greatest strain of physical activity are in the lumbar region, which may be why low back pain is so common.

All your vertebrae have a common structural plan. This includes a vertebral body in front and a number of bony outgrowths, the *pedicles*, the *laminae* and the *articular*, *spinous* and *transverse processes*. These are shown in figure 2. There are however some important variations on this common plan which we will discuss later.

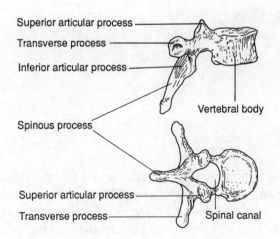

figure 2

Any two vertebrae are joined together in front by the *intervertebral disc* and behind by a pair of small joints, the *posterior vertebral joints*, sometimes known as the *zygoapophyseal joints*. See figure 3.

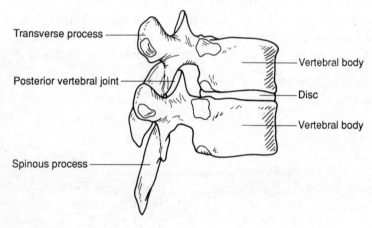

Transverse process

Posterior vertebral joint

Spinous process

Vertebral body

Disc

Vertebral body

figure 3

The intervertebral disc consists of a tough, slightly elastic ring, called the *annulus fibrosus*. This is made in layers, its oblique fibres going alternately one way or the other. The annulus fibrosus is very firmly attached to the edges of the vertebral bodies above and below, and also to the thin cartilaginous end plates of the vertebral bodies. The annulus fibrosus ring contains a jelly-like substance, the *nucleus pulposus*, and plays a part in spinal movement. This is shown in figure 4.

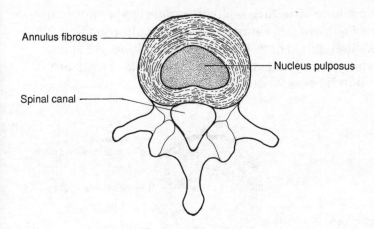

Annulus fibrosus

Nucleus pulposus

Spinal canal

figure 4

The *posterior joints* are much smaller than the disc and are in pairs between the articular processes (the touching, sliding surfaces) of neighbouring vertebrae. The surfaces of these joints are lined with cartilage, which are lubricated by joint fluid, kept in by a joint capsule, in turn supported by a number of small ligaments. This is shown in figure 5.

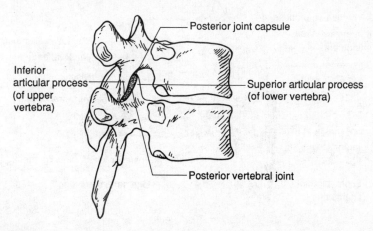

Posterior joint capsule

Inferior articular process (of upper vertebra)

Superior articular process (of lower vertebra)

Posterior vertebral joint

figure 5

The whole structure is given support by a system of seven *ligaments*. Ligaments are strong, fibrous and inelastic bands which hold the bones of the skeleton together and add strength to all the joints. These are shown in figures 6a and 6b.

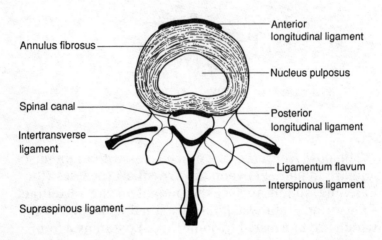

figure 6a

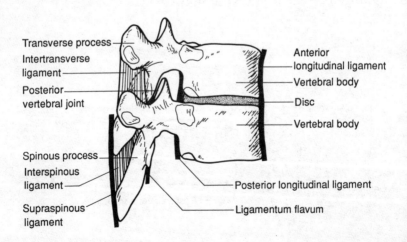

figure 6b

As you can see from figure 2, there is a hole down the middle of the vertebrae, *the spinal canal.* Between each pair of vertebrae there are two holes running sideways, called the *lateral canals.* The spinal canal contains and protects the spinal cord. The lateral canals protect the nerve roots as they branch out from the spinal canal to the rest of the body.

The *spinal cord* is made up of nerve material and is an extension of the brain. It is shorter than the spinal canal and only reaches as far as the first lumbar vertebra. It is protected by a sheath, called the *dura mater.* Within the dura mater the spinal cord floats in the cerebrospinal fluid, which is continuous with the fluid surrounding your brain. From the spinal cord come pairs of nerves, one pair for each vertebral level, each protected by its own sheath of dura. Because the spinal cord is shorter than the bony structure of vertebrae and ends at the first lumbar vertebra, the lower nerve roots extend quite a distance down the spinal canal before they find their own lateral canals and branch down the legs. Over this section the nerves are at risk of interference from anything else which might take up space in the spinal canal or the lateral canals. This, could include a damaged intervertebral disc. See figure 7.

At each end of the spinal column is a ring of bones supporting the limbs. At the top is the *pectoral girdle*, to which our arms are attached. The pectoral girdle is made up of the collar bone and shoulder blades, together with their attachments to the spine. At the base of the spine is the *pelvic girdle* to which our legs are attached. It is made up of the pubic bones and the iliac bones. Figures 8a and 8b show the pectoral girdle and the pelvic girdle respectively.

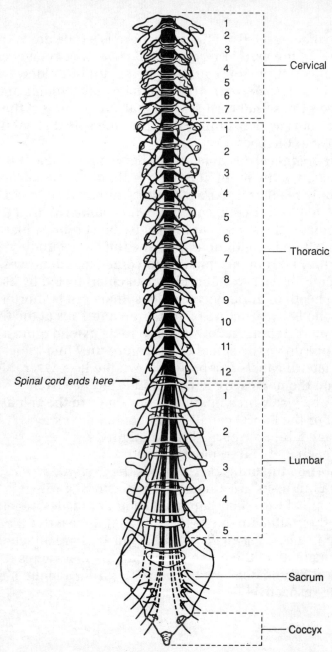

1
2
3
4
5
6
7
— Cervical

1
2
3
4
5
6
7
8
9
10
11
12
— Thoracic

Spinal cord ends here →

1
2
3
4
5
— Lumbar

— Sacrum

— Coccyx

figure 7

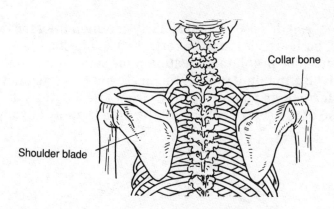

Collar bone

Shoulder blade

figure 8a

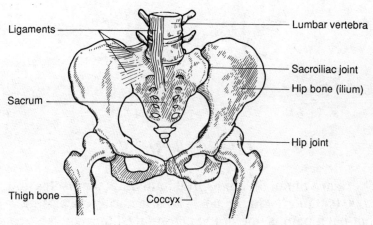

Ligaments

Lumbar vertebra

Sacroiliac joint

Hip bone (ilium)

Sacrum

Hip joint

Thigh bone

Coccyx

figure 8b

The *vertebral arteries* shown in figure 9 are important as the source of blood supply for your brain. You will see that each artery kinks before it enters your skull. Some normal head movements may temporarily block one of these arteries. This has no effect, so long as the other one is not restricted. If, on the other hand, you suffer from arterial disease, which is fairly common in older people, both arteries may be restricted so blockage to one can cause problems. Treatment for some spinal pain may involve manipulation of the neck, but this must not be performed on you if you suffer from arterial disease because of the risk of cutting off the blood supply to your brain!

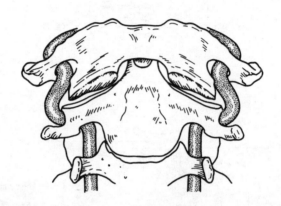

figure 9

CONCLUSION

There are about 50 bones, 100 joints, 1,000 muscles and 1,000,000 nerves in the back, so it is hardly surprising that back pain is one of the commonest human afflictions. There is so much to go wrong! However, we hope that through learning a little bit about the amazing piece of engeering called the back you will come to have some sympathy with the difficulties doctors face when trying to trace the cause of your pain, as well as arming yourself with some of the information necessary to understand what is happening to you. Knowing a bit about the structure of your back will, we hope, lessen your frustration about your situation.

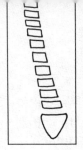

CHAPTER 4

How the back moves

It is not just knowledge of the *structure* of the back which is important for an understanding of back pain, you also need to know a bit about how the back *moves*. Although in real life your whole spine is involved to some extent in any and every movement, for our purposes it is convenient to think of movements as taking place between just two adjacent vertebrae. Two vertebrae and all that separates and connects them are jointly known as the *mobile segment*. This is shown in figure 10.

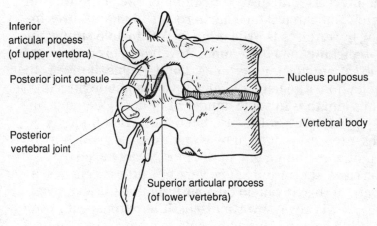

Inferior articular process (of upper vertebra)

Posterior joint capsule

Nucleus pulposus

Posterior vertebral joint

Vertebral body

Superior articular process (of lower vertebra)

figure 10

All the structures in the mobile segment have to move at the same time. Moreover, it is impossible for just one mobile section to move at any time – bits of your back never work in isolation, they all work together.

Pressure on the intervertebral disc

When you think how heavy the upper part of your body is, you can imagine how extreme the forces are in your lower spine. If these forces are too great or too sudden, you are in danger of damaging your back.

Any pressure placed upon a mobile segment will distort the elastic annulus fibrosus of the disc and the nucleus pulposus. Because of the way the annulus fibrosus is built, it will stretch in different directions. This allows one vertebra to press down on the next one, or it can twist slightly on its neighbour, or tip it forwards, backwards or sideways, or it can slide over its neighbour. When you move your back, several of these things may happen at the same time and a problem with any of them may cause pain.

Research has thrown much light on pressures within the intervertebral disc. For example, one of the ways in which you can produce dangerously high pressures in your lower discs is by leaning forward while sitting and then picking up a quite modest weight. This discovery is of great practical importance. For example, it means that a telephonist reaching to pick up a telephone directory at arm's length is in some danger of inflicting damage on his or her spine. It has also been found that high pressures are produced by doing exercises which involve bending, including one of the most widely used exercises, the sit-up! Sadly, very few fitness coaches are aware of this. If you do take part in fitness or exercise classes it is always worth discussing routines with your doctor; he or she should be able to advise you about whether or not they are safe for your back.

The vertebral bodies

When you are sitting or standing the vertebral bodies are the main weight-bearing parts of your spine. Because of their size, shape and arrangement, they play a part in both allowing and limiting movement (see figure 10).

The posterior vertebral joints

The posterior vertebral joints take part in weight-bearing and also in movement of the mobile segment. During movement the surfaces of these joints may be pushed together, pulled apart, angled to each other or slid across each other in one direction or another. All these forms of movement may occur to different degrees every time you change position, and therefore different strains will be put on different parts of your spine. Pain can result if anything interferes with the posterior vertebral joints.

The ligaments

These help to hold the column of vertebrae together, and also play a big part in limiting too much movement, which might otherwise cause damage. When your back is fully bent forwards, your back muscles play no part in maintaining your position, and the ligaments take over this job.

Muscles

Muscle activity can be measured and recorded with great accuracy using highly sensitive devices which register tiny changes in the flow of electric current. Muscles can either contract or relax their contraction, and can do this to very delicately varying degrees. As you might expect, there are hundreds of muscles involved in moving your back, and what they do varies so widely that it is difficult to be certain what any particular muscle is doing at any one time. Some clinicians falsely believe that they can tell what each individual muscle is doing – so be warned! Unfortunately many exercises are based

on outdated ideas as to how muscles work. Again, we
have to stress that sports and fitness coaches may not be
aware of the latest thinking. If you suffer from back pain,
but want to maintain your fitness, always ask a doctor to
comment on your routines.

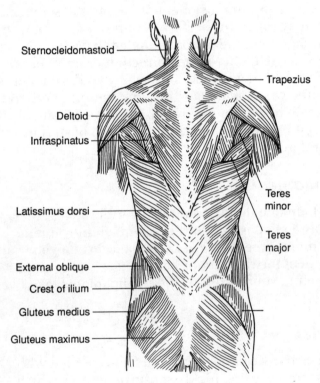

The main muscles of the back

Tendons

These are the ropes which attach your muscles to bones.
If you contract a muscle, it will pull through its tendons,
bringing the points of bony attachment nearer together.
If there is a joint between the two bones the muscle is
attached to, then such a pull will move that joint. It may

be stopped from moving, if another opposing muscle contracts at the same time, or if there is a physical obstruction to movement. But the muscular pull is always transmitted through your tendons.

The spinous and transverse processes

The spinous and transverse processes act as levers, to which muscles are attached by their tendons and through which they pull and relax when you move or maintain your posture. We say *pull* or *relax*, because any movement requires some muscles to pull, while others relax. If all muscles pulled together, the result would be that your spine stiffened and movement was prevented.

CONCLUSION

Next time you bend forward, pick up a book, look to your side, walk upstairs or perform any simple, everyday activity, think of all the processes taking place in your back – and think of all the things that can go wrong. When you remember how complex the back is, and how complex the movement within it, it is surprising back pain is not even more common!

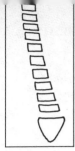

CHAPTER 5

Pain: all in the mind?

One of the frustrating things about back pain is that causes are so difficult to pin down and completely effective treatments are fairly rare. This means that back problems can drag on for years; you may have to see a succession of advisers and specialists, none of whom can provide an effective solution. These factors may lead people to accuse you of malingering – a charge which can be difficult to answer, especially if it comes from unsympathetic colleagues who think you are not pulling your weight at work, or if the accusation is made by your boss. If you are accused of malingering, stick to your guns. You could give your detractors a copy of this book; by reading it they might come to understand the complexity of the problems you face and thus become more understanding towards you.

If you have suffered from back pain for a long time and cannot get relief, you may even come to believe that it's all in your mind – that you are going mad and imaging the pain. These suspicions can be even more depressing

Are psychological factors important in back pain? Well, they are certainly involved in our experience of pain. It is now recognised that pain is a complex experience with evidence confirming that it involves variation in several factors, dependent upon ever changing states, including mental states, continuously influenced by a multitude of enviromental, perceptual, emotional and bodily stimulae. Psychology is inevitably involved with our experience of pain.

than other people's accusations of malingering – do not give way to them. Descartes said *I think therefore I am*; a similar argument can be used when it comes to pain – *if you think you are in pain, then you are in pain.* Remember this argument next time you think you might be going mad and imagining the pain.

THINKING ABOUT PAIN

How pain is felt (or not)

Neurology is the study of nerves. The neurology of pain is very complicated, but fascinating. Its study offers rich rewards in a better understanding of how we feel pain – or why, in some cases, we don't. *Articular neurology* is the study of the nerve supply to joints and was a neglected field of study until a few years ago. It has now revealed a great deal about how pain is felt and which structures it may come from. You will only feel pain if certain nerve endings, *nociceptors*, are stimulated. Stimulation may be chemical or mechanical. Chemical stimulation may arise in conditions where dangerous substances build up to sufficient levels in the body. The causes of these conditions include inflammatory disease like rheumatoid arthritis. Chemical stimulation can also arise if your tissues are deprived of oxygen – this explains the cramp-like pains felt after too much exercise.

The other way of stimulating nerve endings is mechanical – pricking, pressing, moving, etc. Everyone knows the pain of accidentally pricking a finger or pinching it in the door, and many back pain sufferers know how dramatically painful it may be to rick the back.

When there is either chemical or mechanical stimulation of the nociceptors they at once fire off messages through the nerves into the spinal cord. But other messages are also constantly coming into the spinal cord. So we have a situation in which messages from both *nociceptors* (pain messages) and messages from *mechanoceptors* (position messages) are both competing to be transferred via the nerves in the spinal cord to the brain. If there are enough messages from the mechanoceptors, those from the nociceptors will not 'get through the gate' and no pain will be felt. This explains why people may not feel the pain from a serious injury until quite some time after the injury was inflicted – the pain messages from the site of the injury are competing with other messages being transmitted up the spinal cord and the brain refuses to 'let them through the gate'.

> The consequences of emotion on pain have been known for hundreds of years. In 1580 Montaigne wrote 'we feel the nick of the barber's razor more keenly than ten sword wounds received in the heat of battle'. But of course it is only recently that we have been able to give a scientific explanation of the phenomenon.

There are at least three treatments of back pain which make use of the fact that the brain will not let pain messages 'through the gate', so that pain will not be felt, if there are enough messages of other sorts competing to be let through. They are:

- Massage – an ancient treatment, much relied on by alternative practitioners.
- Manipulation – another ancient treatment widely used by osteopaths, chiropractors and an increasing number of doctors and physiotherapists.
- Transcutaneous electrical nerve stimulation (TENS) – a very recent treatment indeed, usually only offered in hospitals but machines for use at home are available.

We will discuss these three treatments in chapter 8.

How you feel about your pain

The psychologist uses the term *affect* to describe the way you feel about pain. The longer your pain persists, the more likely you will become depressed, afraid and irritable. These changes affect those around you – your family, friends, employer and colleagues. The longer the pain lasts, the more likely is it that you will become seriously depressed. Ten per cent of people attending pain clinics are found to have classic symptoms of depressive illness. (For more about pain clinics see page 107.) If you are not depressed, we do not want to alarm you, but we think that 'forewarned is forearmed'. If you recognise depression as a possible consequence of pain, you may feel better able to approach a doctor for help, if you suspect you are becoming a victim. If you have suffered depression, or are suffering pain-related depression now, we hope that you will draw some comfort from the fact that you are not alone. If you have not discussed depression with a doctor, we would urge you to do so.

How you understand your pain

The psychologists call the way you understand your pain *cognition* and it is also of great importance when thinking about pain. The classic example of this is the comparison of the understanding of wounds suffered by soldiers in battle and by civilians in accidents. There are striking differences in the way these two groups of people react to their injuries. This is because a battle wound for the soldier means escape from a life-threatening situation and a return home, whereas injury for the civilian presents a threat to his comfortable life. The two groups understand their wounds in different ways so react differently to them.

What you do because of your pain

Pain behaviour is what you actually *do* because of your pain. For example, how many tablets you take; how much time you spend in bed; how your pain affects your ability to do jobs both at home and at work; and how you get on with those around you. (You may find pain makes you irritable towards loved ones, but explain to them you are bad-tempered because of your back, not because of them!)

Pain may lead you to form habits, which may be either good or bad. Habits are of course a form of behaviour. It would be a good habit to get into a regular exercise routine as research has shown that people who exercise make fewer complaints about back pain than people who never exercise. Ask your doctor for a safe routine. It would be a bad habit to start taking too many pain-killers as research shows that people who take pain-killers are prescribed more drugs than other people when they are admitted to hospital – since drugs may have long-term side-effects it is often best to try to avoid them.

CONCLUSION

When thinking about back pain it is impossible to divorce psychological factors from physical ones – the mind and the body interact together to produce the complex phenomenon we call *pain*. Most doctors understand this, but occasionally a doctor might say that your pain is all in your mind – usually because his or her suggested therapy is not working. This chapter should have given you the ammunition to convince your doctor that they are being short-sighted if they accuse you of imagining it all. In this situation, do not blame your doctor; doctors' training is not geared up to managing pain. It is the medical education system that is at fault – not individual doctors.

CHAPTER 6

Diagnosis

What has already been said about the many causes of back pain (chapter 2) and the interplay of physical and psychological factors (chapter 5) partly explains why doctors find reaching a confident diagnosis of back pain so difficult. In fact it is harder than we have already suggested; there are three further complicating factors:

- What is known as the *subject report*. When you describe your pain to a doctor, your description is subjective. It relies on your own individual experience, your own emotional involvement with your pain and your own understanding of it. Such subjective reports are hard to accommodate in the objective world of science because general conclusions cannot be drawn from them. The unavoidable subjectivity of your reports makes diagnosis very difficult.
- What is known as *referred pain*. Problems with your back do not necessarily result in back pain; the pain can be referred to almost any other part of your body. Pain referral is unpredictable and therefore bedevils diagnosis. We discuss pain referral further in the next chapter.
- Even if problems with your back are felt as pain in your back, it is almost always impossible to say precisely where in the spine your pain originates because nociceptors (pain signalling nerves, see chapter 5) are present in the great majority of spinal tissues, any one of which could be the source of pain, and because all the different parts of your back are so

closely bound up with one another in terms of both structure and function.

All this means that you must be very wary of anybody who comes up with an immediate and confident diagnosis of your problem. Such a person may be banging a drum for a possibly mistaken theory of pain and offer you very specific advice and a limited range of treatments. Occasionally you may meet such an overconfident attitude from someone practising one of the vast range of alternative and complementary therapies, and the orthodox members of our profession are certainly not immune. The factors outlined above also give you further ammunition against those who might accuse you of malingering. Just because doctors cannot give you a diagnosis does not mean that nothing is the matter, it just indicates the complexity of the problem.

> 'The range of labels used in connection with back pain is a fair reflection of medical ignorance and factional interest.'
> Professor Anderson, a specialist at Guy's Hospital, London University, with a particular interest in backs.

Given the problems, you may ask why anybody ever bothers to examine your back! The answer is twofold. Firstly, physical examination can reveal the spinal level which is abnormal, allowing one of the many local treatments to be targeted to it to give some degree of relief. (Spinal level simply means the level of each vertebral body.) Secondly, physical examination allows doctors to review the progress of treatment, as improvements in the patient's condition will often be picked up.

Doctors use two sorts of tests when examining your back, those involving light touch and those involving firm pressure. We will now discuss each of these in turn.

Light pressure tests

SKIN PINCHING TEST

This is used to find areas of your skin which cause you pain if pinched quite lightly. Pinching harder is not helpful. Often your doctor will find a level where you say 'ow' on one side of your spine and not on the other. This may be an illustration of *referred tenderness*. Referred tenderness means that the pain is produced as a result of a disorder elsewhere and an appropriate local treatment may be prescribed.

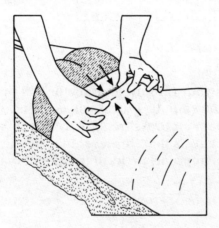

MUSCLE TONE TEST

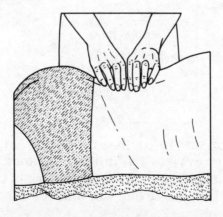

In this test doctors are looking for areas where your muscle tone is greater than elsewhere. What is meant by increased muscle tone is a feeling of greater resistance to pressure, again finding a site of increased muscle tone can lead to a local treatment being prescribed.

TENDERNESS TEST
This involves pressing really quite firmly, in a search for tender spots or *trigger points*. These are painful, tender knobs in the soft tissues, such as muscle, and may be further examples of referred tenderness, only this time deeper than in the skin pinching test.

Deep pressure tests

DIRECT PRESSURE
As you lie on your tummy your doctor will press directly down on to the spinous process of each vertebra in turn, looking for pain on pressure. If there is pain at one point or level, it suggests that this level may be the source of your pain. An appropriate local treatment may then be prescribed.

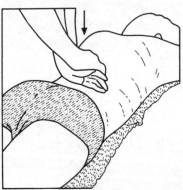

PRESSING EACH VERTEBRAL SPINOUS PROCESS SIDEWAYS
Pressing sideways on each vertebral spinous process tends to twist each vertebra to left and right between its neighbours. If pressing one way and not the other causes

pain at any point or level, it suggests that what is wrong with you is being stretched or compressed by one movement, and not by the other. So we are getting nearer to discovering *where* you have something wrong, if not necessarily to knowing what to do about it.

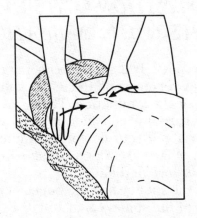

PRESSING DOWN OVER EACH POSTERIOR VERTEBRAL JOINT
This test involves pressing down on each posterior vertebral joint. These joints lie on either side of the

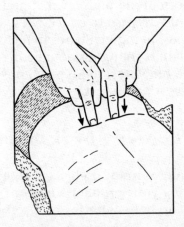

spinous processes. The test aims to discover if you have one or more posterior joints which is tender. If you do, it suggests we may have found the source of the pain and may be able to prescribe a local treatment.

EXAMINATION OTHER THAN PHYSICAL EXAMINATION

Occasionally, especially if surgery is being considered, your doctor may recommend the use of a diagnostic tool other than physical examination. The use of such tools should be very carefully considered, as they are not always appropriate. If your doctor recommends X-rays or laboratory test, make sure that he or she fully explains the intended purpose of them.

X-rays show the shadows of the bones in detail. The size and shape of the spinal canal and its exits can be assessed. The discs do not show up, only the spaces they occupy. X-rays can show a cracked or fractured vertebra and reveal degenerative changes and signs of abnormalities in the vertebrae. 'Soft' tissues, such as discs, muscles and ligaments, do not show up. However, the Royal College of Radiographers has recently expressed concern at the high level of non-essential X-rays, so it would be wise to check with your clinician that X-rays you are being given are in fact necessary.

If your back pain is thought *not* to be mechanical, you may be offered a blood test to help diagnosis, and, of course, other investigations, if deemed necessary.

ASSESSING PAIN BEHAVIOUR

It is not only changes in local physical signs that are useful in assessing your problem and your progress. A record of your pain behaviour is also useful. How often

MUSCULOSKELETAL CASE ANALYSIS SHEET

Patient's name: .... Serial no: ....

Address: .... Phone: ....

.... Insurance: ....

Date of birth: / / Male .... Female ....

Contraindications: Fracture ..... Neoplasm ..... Scheuermann ..... A/spondylitis .....
Polymyalgia ..... Osteoporosis ..... Rh. A. of neck ..... Basilar insuff ..... Grisel .....
Myelopathy ..... Sphincter problems ...... Saddle anaesthesia .....

HISTORY - Present episode

Subject report

		/ /		/ /		/ /	
		L	R	L	R	L	R
Pain -	Site						
	Radiation						
	Intensity						
	Duration						
	Worsened by						
	Improved by						

Altered sensation

	P & N						
	Numbness						

Activities of daily living

	Hoovering						
	Bedmaking						
	Ablutions						
	Cooking						
	Ironing						
	Putting on socks						
	Shopping						
	Gardening						
	Sports						
	Sitting at desk						
	Other work						
	Road/rail travel						
	Air travel						

Pain behaviour

	Pill taking habit						
	Other treatment						
	Hours bed per 24						
	Forced absenteeism						
	Litigation pending						

Previous episodes

Year .... Site .... Duration in Days ...... Weeks ...... Months ......

Therapy .... Outcome ....

Year .... Site .... Duration in Days ...... Weeks ...... Months ......

Therapy .... Outcome ....

Relevant medical history ....

....

Affect ....

you take pain-killers, retire to bed, alter your daily routine or complain to your friends about your back can help doctors to build up a useful profile to be used in deciding your treatment. We include on page 35 part of a record sheet which doctors might use to monitor your pain behaviour.

A precise record of changes in your pain behaviour can give us a better idea of how you are getting on than any other. The advantage of this, compared with your 'subject report', is that we can measure these changes, even though we cannot measure pain. This can be encouraging for you, proving changes have taken place when you thought you were getting nowhere.

Cautionary note

In this chapter we have given an account of how *we* proceed, but there are other people who have different ideas and who go about assessment in different ways. Indeed, there are almost as many methods of assessment as there are people interested in back pain. The point we are making is that the absence of a diagnosis is not a cause for despair. On the contrary, it means that you will not be shackled by a label which, by its false certainty, may dominate the treatment you are given, the advice you receive, and indeed your whole life. If your back pain is not diagnosed precisely, a flexible approach to both treatment and advice is the only approach.

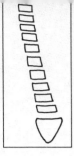

CHAPTER 7

The back and the whole body

There are two facts about the spine and pain which may confuse you:

- Problems in the spine can lead to pain in almost any part of the body – this is the phenomenon of referred pain mentioned in the last chapter.
- Problems in the spine can result in symptoms which may be confused with the symptoms of a range of diseases, including heart and abdominal complaints.

In this chapter we will explore the effects problems with your back can have on other parts of your body.

Headaches and 'migraines'

It has been shown that perhaps as many as one-in-three headaches originate in the neck. This means that, if you suffer from frequent headaches and need to see your doctor about the problem, you should ask to have your neck examined. The neck often causes one-sided headache, which may be misdiagnosed as *migraine*. Migraine is a miserable complaint. If you suffer from it ask your

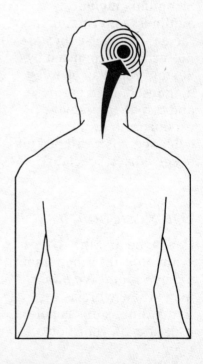

doctor to look at your neck.
If positive local signs are
found, he or she might
then be able to
recommend treatments.

Bizarre symptoms of spinal origin

These are peculiar
symptoms you might not
normally expect to come
from your spine. They are
not uncommon and often
confuse medics, for they
may suggest ear, nose and
throat conditions.
Symptoms include
giddiness and ringing in
the ears. Because they are
not widely recognised by
doctors you may be mis-
diagnosed. If an ear nose
and throat assessment
produces no positive
evidence it is worth asking
to see a back specialist.

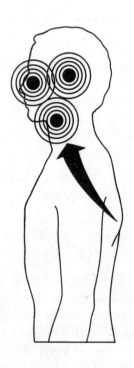

Whiplash injuries

Headache and the
symptoms described under
Bizarre spinal symptoms
may follow whiplash
injury. But as this is not
well known, your neck

may not be examined, even if whiplash is established. You may be considered to be neurotic or to be suffering from 'post-traumatic neurosis' if you continue to complain. This is unfortunate, for several different treatments applied to the neck might alleviate your pain. If you feel run-down after a whiplash injury, but there seems to be no cause of your aches and pains, again ask to see a back specialist.

Referral of pain to the shoulder and arm

This is not uncommon with neck problems and it can be a source of confusion. Referred tenderness can produce physical signs, which, if the spine is not examined, may indicate conditions such as tennis elbow or the carpal tunnel syndrome (a condition that causes pain/altered sensations in the hand), when in fact the symptoms are really caused by problems in the spine.

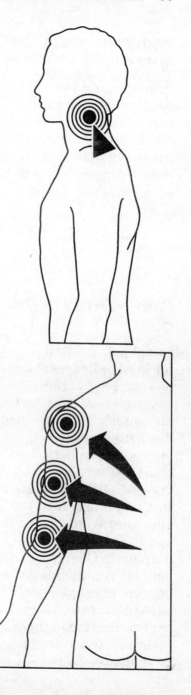

Pain referred to the upper back

Pain between your shoulder blades often comes from your neck. If this is not considered, treatment may well prove unsatisfactory, as it will be targeted at the wrong place.

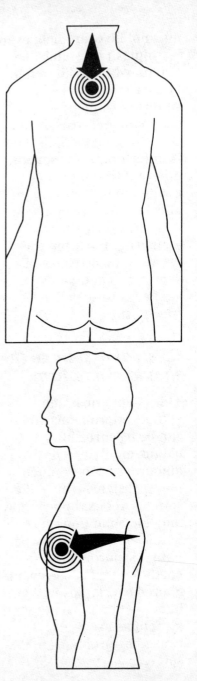

Pain referred to the chest

Spinal pain is often referred to the chest and this can have serious consequences for you. If the spine is not examined, this pain may be interpreted as indicating heart disease. This is unnecessarily upsetting for you, and it may lead you to alter your whole way of life. In one university hospital in Denmark, patients admitted because of acute chest pain were studied over two years. In twenty per cent of them their pain was traced to their spines.

Pain referred to the abdomen

Abdominal pain is not often in fact associated with the spine, although the spine may be the source of the problem. Misdiagnosis can lead to unnecessary abdominal investigations, even to surgery. In one instance a patient's abdomen had been operated on no fewer than three times, when in fact his pain arose from problems with his spine.

Pain referred to the low back

Again this is not well understood and it is not unusual for patients to receive extensive treatment to the lumbar spine, even surgery, when the pain really arises higher up the back.

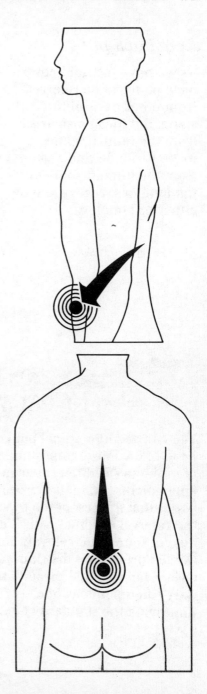

Low back pain

As we have just said, low back pain can be referred from other parts of the spine. But it can also arise from the lumbar spine itself. It can be referred from the lumbar spine to the buttocks, coccyx and to either or both legs.

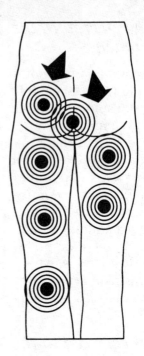

CONCLUSION

You can see how spinal pain can indeed be felt from head to toe. More important, it can confuse the diagnosis of problems as different as migraine, heart disease and appendicitis. And it is *very* common. The bad news for you is that at present too few doctors know much about the referral of spinal pain. The good news is that a great deal of sound and relevant information does now exist; the big problem is distributing it. Happily, it is becoming easier, for example through the setting up of the Primary Care Rheumatology Society (the PCR), which aims at improving the standard of general practice in this field.

CHAPTER 8

Treatments that may help

We have already seen that it is difficult to find the cause of a back pain problem and difficult to give an accurate diagnosis. This means that it is also difficult to plan treatment – the honest truth is that treatment is often a matter of trial and error! You should remember this if you are contemplating major treatment such as surgery. However, it is still worth exploring what treatments are available, and how they work. The treatments we review and the chart we provide show that quite how they work, and indeed whether they will work, either in the short term or in the long term, is often largely unknown. But the gate theory does partly explain the effectiveness of some treatments. You will remember that input into the spinal cord from the mechanoceptors can inhibit input from the nociceptors. What this means is that, if you have enough input from mechanical stimulation, you can stop pain being felt. This helps explain the effectiveness of massage, manipulation and transcutaneous nerve stimulation.

Any treatment you receive may affect you in several ways so do not accept defeat if one or two different treatments fail to help you. It is too easy to become depressed. 'Prudent optimism' should be your slogan! There are many treatments for back pain. Which treatment you are offered will depend largely on the person you go to for help. In chapter 9 we discuss some groups of people who may help you. Here we look at a number of treatments you may be offered in rather the same way, usually answering the following five questions:

- How do you get the treatment?
- Who is likely to give the treatment?
- Will the treatment help you?
- Will the treatment hurt?
- Can the treatment do any harm?

Analgesics (pain-killers)

How do you get them? Either over the counter or prescribed by your doctor. There are literally hundreds of easily available pain-killers, including aspirin and paracetamol.

Will they help you? This will vary from drug to drug, from person to person and from problem to problem. The only way to find the answer is by trial and error.

Can they do you any harm? Unhappily, they can, for all of them could have some dangers. Therefore it is important for you to use them as little as you can. You must take them only when really necessary to relieve your pain, and under no circumstances take them for the sake of it. This is of the greatest importance.

Anti-inflammatory drugs

As their name suggests this class of drugs reduces inflammation and thus may help reduce your pain. Normally they are available through your doctor. Comments on the analgesics apply equally to this group. Nurofen is widely available over the counter.

Anti-depressants

How do you get them? On prescription from your doctor.

Who is likely to give them? You should take them as directed by your doctor. They will have good reasons for prescribing these drugs, and you must keep to the directions given.

Will they help you? They are used widely, but there is little evidence that this is justified. They should come a long way down the list of treatments offered to you. But ten per cent of patients seen at pain clinics are depressed and need anti-depressant treatment.

Can they do any harm? Yes. You can become addicted to the anti-depressants, which is one reason why you must only take them as directed.

Narcotic drugs

These are very strong pain-killers.

How do you get them? They will be prescribed by a doctor. These are used only when your pain is severe.

Will they help you? Very likely, yes. Narcotic drugs are the most effective pain-killers of all.

Can they do you any harm? YES. The risks of addiction are very serious. For this reason their supply is strictly controlled, and doctors are very reluctant to prescribe them. However bad your back problem may be, it is very dangerous for you to obtain these drugs on the open market.

Tranquillisers

These are widely prescribed today, often without good cause, and they share the same problems as the anti-depressants.

Bedrest

How do you get it? Most often you go to bed, encouraged by your family or by your doctor. Less frequently you may have this thrust upon you in hospital.

Do not worry too much about the type of mattress you lie on; the most important point is to be comfortable.

Will it help you? In a very severe, acute attack, it may well be the only thing you can do, and it will certainly seem to help you in the short term.

Can it do any harm? It has recently (1986) been shown that prolonged bedrest has no advantage over early mobilisation, and may itself produce problems, including pain behaviour. Therefore, doctors nowadays should think twice before recommending bed rest.

Heat and cold

You may find either heat or cold a help. So, with a hot water bottle and a refrigerator, there is nothing to stop you becoming an excellent therapist! The important point here is that you must give enough time to either treatment. It should last at least 20 minutes and should be repeated at least once a day. Heat or cold should be applied directly to the painful area – if you are at home you might need to ask for help. A useful way of applying cold is with a packet of frozen peas – just the right sort of size, and it can be easily moulded to your shape. A hot water bottle wrapped in a towel is the best way of applying heat.

How do you get heat and cold treatments? At home, or in a physiotherapy department.

Will they help? Quite likely, yes. Give them a trial. (Remember trial and error is an important ingredient of back paint treatment.)

Will they hurt? Not unless you overdo them and either burn yourself, or get frostbite!

Electrical treatments

These include shortwave diathermy (SWD), ultrasound, interferential therapy and a number of rather similar treatments.

How do you get them? Usually from a physiotherapist, but a number of other groups use them, such as osteopaths, chiropractors, and those attached to sports clinics and fitness clubs.

Will they help you? They may, but there is no way of telling beforehand – again, it's a case of trial and error.

Will they hurt? They should not but they may, if wrongly used, and you should certainly tell your clinician if you feel pain during the treatment.

Can they do any harm? Only if incorrectly used. Some years ago it was wrongly thought that the way they worked was understood. Since then doctors have realised they *don't* know how these treatments work and they have lost standing in the eyes of some and are less favoured.

Collars and corsets

How do you get them? Usually on prescription, but there is nothing to stop you buying them direct from suppliers; many types are available.

Will they help you? They may. The only way to find out is to try them.

Will they hurt? They should not, but if they do, take them off at once.

Can they do any harm? Not much, but, if they are *not* helping you, you may continue to use them when you might better try another form of treatment.

Traction

This is a well-known treatment which is currently out of favour because it has not been shown to be better than any other. On the other hand, it certainly has its successes.

How do you get it? Usually through referral by your doctor to a physiotherapist.

Will it help you? Yes, quite often, but it is not possible to predict who will be helped.

Will it hurt? It should not. If it does tell the physiotherapist to stop.

Can it do any harm? Not if you stop when it hurts! It is possible to give yourself traction at home, using a simple apparatus. You may find this helpful, but you should consult your doctor first.

Auto suspension

How do you get it? Preferably, on the advice of your doctor, though you could buy a machine yourself.

Will it help you? It may or may not; try it and see.

Will it hurt? Possibly. If it does, stop using it at once.

Can it do you any harm? Those machines that tip you up may cause appreciable discomfort. So generally speaking, the answer is, not if you stop when it hurts. There is no proof that being suspended upside-down is any better for you than ordinary traction, where you stay the right way up.

Massage and manipulation

We group these two treatments together because they work in more or less the same way. That is, they stimulate the mechanoceptors, preventing the nociceptors from sending pain messages to the brain.

How do you get massage and manipulation? You could ask a friend or partner to give you a massage, or you have a professional massage. If you know someone who uses aromatherapy oils in conjunction with massage, receiving treatment from them could be very pleasant, even if not especially effective! Your doctor, an osteopath or a chiropractor may recommend manipulation.

Will they help you? Very often, yes. But be careful if undergoing massage from someone lacking medical qualifications.

Will they hurt? They should not. If they do, more than a very little, you should tell your chosen massager or manipulator to stop.

Can they do any harm? Damage from either massage or manipulation is very rare, but this needs a little discussion. If you suffer from 'numb bum', a condition where there may be pressure on the nerves supplying the bladder, or become giddy when standing up or turning sharply, manipulation could be very dangerous for you. There are a number of diseases in which manipulation should never be used, when the blood supply to the brain could be cut off. The safest way to avoid trouble is to get a properly qualified opinion, from whatever source. The only possible harm from massage is that, if it is very rough, it may produce bruising.

We though it appropriate here to reproduce an article from *The Independent on Sunday*, 9 May 1993.

Manipulation and massage

FROM ancient times, charismatic popular healers have laid their hands on a sick person's body while more orthodox practitioners have preferred to keep body contact to a minimum. For hundreds of years in Britain, surgeons – who set broken bones and dealt with wounds and abscesses – were regarded as socially inferior to physicians, who made their diagnosis at a distance. Surgeons and physicians have long since made up their differences, but body contact with patients is still seen by many doctors as being on the fringe of mainstream scientific medicine.

The main exception is the manipulation used by orthopaedic surgeons to restore damaged bones and joints to a normal position. This is a continuation of a long tradition: in the past, before anaesthetics and X-rays, skilled bonesetters became famous for their ability to use their hands to discover how to reposition broken bones so that they would heal without deformity. This repositioning is just as important today, though X-rays have made it easier, and rapid healing depends on accurate positioning of the bone fragments. Manipula-tion of a dislocated joint is another skilled procedure; it is not just a matter of putting the bones back into place, but of doing so without causing any further damage to ligaments.

It is manipulation of the spine that is the really controversial issue. The 33 bones of the spinal column are joined together by tough cartilage discs, and they also have small facet joints which allow the spine to bend, twist and rotate. In the 19th century, the founders of osteopathy and chiropractic developed whole theories of medicine based on the belief that many diseases of the digestion, heart and lungs were due to subtle small faults in the alignment of the spinal bones. These misalignments were thought to interfere with the nerves and blood vessels, and so disturb the general health. Both systems were based on the belief that spine manipulation could restore normal health.

Nowadays, osteopaths and chiropractors make less wide-ranging claims. But they still assert that the health of many people can be improved by putting their spines back into the correct healthy position. Mainstream doctors agree that many people with backache benefit from having spines massaged and manipulated, freeing joints and encouraging an optimum posture. Research has shown that people with back pain recover more quickly following manipulation than when simply told to rest in bed and take pain-relieving tablets. Osteopathy and chiropractic are regaining status and becoming more popular as victims of backache discover the benefits of therepeutic manipulation.

Massage, like manipulation, may be orthodox or alternative. Orthodox is prescribed by doctors and carried out by physiotherapists, while a whole range of massage therapies in the private sector are claimed to enhance health. Massage is said to increase the blood to the muscles, to loosen up tense muscles and ligaments, and to help stiff joints move. Just why massage makes most people feel better is not at all clear. Touch seems to have calming, relaxing, life-enhancing properties. Doctors who remain aloof from physical contact with patients are denying them one of the oldest ingredients of the healing process.

Dr Tony Smith

Local anaesthetic injections

How do you get them? At the hands of a doctor.

Who will give them? Your doctor (*not* a nurse or paramedic) will give you your injection. Local anaesthetic injections for back pain, may be given at many different sites, depending on the physical signs that are found during examination.

Will they help you? Very likely, yes, although sometimes only in the short term as the effect may wear off after a few hours.

Will they hurt? Any injection hurts, but remember that the injection may well help to get rid of a much greater pain.

Can they do any harm? Not in the hands of a properly trained doctor.

Steroid injections

Steroids are often used in conjunction with local anaesthetics, but they may be given on their own.

Similar remarks apply to steroid injections as to local anaesthetic injections. Many people have expressed fear about the use of steroid drugs, probably fuelled by the media reports about the use of steroids by athletes and sportsmen. Be reassured that, used properly, these drugs may be of great benefit and have none of the nasty side effects so often attributed to them.

Epidural injections

You may meet these in two different forms. One, the *caudal epidural*, is given via your *sacral hiatus* (a hole in your sacrum, convenient for injection). This is a relatively simple injection in general practice, with the same problems and advantages as discussed under local anaesthetic injections. *Lumbar epidural injections* can be very helpful, but they must only be given in hospital. Lumbar epidural injections are often given to women in labour.

Transcutaneous nerve stimulation (TENS)

So far as is known, this stimulation works in very much the same way as do massage and manipulation. TENS involves electrical stimulation of the mechanoceptor nerve fibres using needle electrodes through the skin thus blocking pain perception in the spinal cord.

How do you get it? Usually through a doctor. However, you can buy a machine and administer TENS at home. You may be able to borrow a machine, to give it a trial before buying one. Consult your doctor before you administer TENS at home. He or she is likely to refer you to a Pain Clinic as the next stage.

Will it help? Quite likely. It is well worth trying, if you have chronic pain.

Will it hurt? No – unless you turn it up too high! Then it may still work, as a form of 'hyperstimulation'. That is, it works like acupuncture and will not do you any harm.

Acupuncture and acupressure

Acupuncture is the Oriental method for relieving pain using fine needles inserted at specific points to stimulate nerve impulses. Acupressure does not use needles and can be practised at home – precise finger pressure is applied to the same spots where the acupuncturist inserts needles.

How do you get it? Your doctor may suggest acupuncture, or provide it, though usually you will have to find an alternative practitioner. You usually administer acupressure to yourself.

Who will provide it? Many people offer acupuncture, so make sure they have some sort of qualification and are experienced in its use. You can contact the Natural Medicine Society to find out about acupuncture and other complementary therapies.

Will they help you? Often, yes, so they are well worth a try, if other treatments have failed.

Will they hurt? Acupuncture may hurt a little; acupressure does not hurt at all.

Can they do any harm? In the hands of an experienced, properly trained person acupuncture will do no harm. Try to check hygiene standards; all reputable practitioners will use sterile needles, discarded after use.

Orthodox medical scientists have now established that you can get substantial relief of pain from the insertion of a hypodermic needle into a suitable place without any injection. Although the *placebo effect* can not be discounted, it appears that the results are better than could be expected from this alone. (The placebo effect occurs when you get relief from something without medical properties because you *believe* you will get relief from the treatment.) The only rational explanation is that every injection involves an element of acupuncture. So, if your doctor suggests this approach, give it a try.

Rhizolysis and rhizotomy

These are surgical procedures which involve killing some of your nerve endings. (See appendix 4.)

How do you get them? By referral by your doctor.

Who will give them? A hospital specialist.

Will they help you? They may.

Will they hurt? Like all surgical procedures, they may leave you feeling a bit sore.

Will they do any harm? Not if given by a properly qualified person.

Nerve root surgery

This may be a last ditch treatment, when pain has become unbearable, and no way has been found to stop it. It involves surgery to cut the nerve supply to the offending part.

How do you get it? By referral to hospital.

Who will give it? A hospital specialist.

Will it help? Often, yes – since nerves are severed, pain messages cannot be transmitted to the brain.

Will it hurt? All surgery involves some pain.

Will it do any harm? It may do, because *all* major surgery carries risks which is why this is a last resort, not to be undertaken lightly.

Disc surgery

This is surgery to remove disc material which may be causing your pain. It has the same problems and potential as has nerve root surgery. It is a major procedure and should never be undertaken lightly.

Chemonucleolysis

This is a rare treatment. Chemonucleolysis is an injection into the middle of one of your intervertebral discs and is intended to dissolve the nucleus pulposus. It is done under X-ray control, and under an anaesthetic.

How do you get it? At the hands of one of the few

doctors who use this form of treatment, on referral by your own doctor.

Will it help you? It may do. As yet not a great deal is known about the long-term results, and it must be said that it has enjoyed a rather stormy passage since its introduction. Arguments have raged as to its efficacy and its safety.

Sclerosant therapy

This has been used widely in the past, but it is currently out of fashion for it has no clear advantage over other treatments and is very painful. It involves the injection of irritant solutions aimed at tightening up ligaments thought to be slack.

Hypnosis

This has been much studied, particularly in the relief of dental pain, where it has proved very useful. Hypnosis has been found to be less useful in relieving back pain. It is thought that this may be because the cause of back pain is usually not clear, so hypnotic suggestion cannot be used to overcome it. However, it is still worth a try.

How do you get it? Usually under your own steam, although your doctor may refer you to a hypnotherapist. Increasingly, doctors use this form of therapy themselves, for example to help people give up smoking.

Who will provide it? Anybody can claim to offer hypnotherapy, so make sure your hypnotherapist is reputable – try and get some personal recommendations from other people who have used his or her services. Since there have recently been several scare stories about women being abused whilst hypnotised, it is probably worth asking your doctor to recommend a GP who offers the service.

Will it help you? Quite likely, but it is unpredictable.

Will it hurt? No.

Can it do any harm? Baldly, yes. This is because you may react violently to it. If you do, and no one can tell in advance, this then can only be handled by a properly trained, experienced therapist. So you must check on this before you get involved.

Biofeedback and relaxation response

These are psychotherapies and because they act in a similar way, we treat these two together.

How do you get them? Usually by referral from your doctor but they are also available from complementary practitioners.

Who will give them? Either hospital staff or you may use them on your own or in classes.

Biofeedback and relaxation response may help, will not hurt and will not do any harm.

Behavioural therapy and cognitive behavioural therapy

Again because of their similarity, we treat these two therapies together. They both involve counselling and are concerned with the psychological aspects of pain.

How do you get them? By referral by your doctor.

Who will give them? A hospital specialist.

Will they help? Often, yes. They are particularly useful for those of you with really chronic pain, and they are intended to improve the quality of life, rather than to relieve your pain.

Psychotherapy and counselling

Private psychotherapists and counsellors, who will try to uncover any emotional causes of your pain, mainly through question and answer sessions, may also help you to come to terms with your back pain. Contact the umbrella organisations and the British Psychotherapy Association for advice and information (see appendix 4).

Exercises

Exercises form the commonest group of physical treatments offered to you if you have back pain, though, it has never been proved that they have any direct effect in prevention or treatment. Neither has it been proved that weak muscles increase your chance of developing back pain. On the other hand, it has been shown that exercises which involve a great deal of movement, such as touching your toes, can increase the pressure inside your discs, which may actually cause trouble for you. Perhaps surprisingly, your tummy muscles can take some of the load off your spine, so trying to strengthen these makes sense. Once again, there are a lot of conflicting opinions, none of which has so far been shown to be true! Again, our advice has to be for you to be wary of dogmatic statements and to go for what you find helps, always remembering to avoid excessive movements. Once more, safety is more important for you than imagined efficacy. In the light of this, we describe and illustrate just two simple back exercises (in appendix 2); these can do no harm and you may find them helpful.

TREATMENTS TABLE

The following table summarises the information provided in this chapter. In the *cost* column 'A' means 'cheap', 'B' means 'moderate' and 'C' means 'expensive'. The *time* column refers to how long the treatment takes to start having an effect. Column 'A' means 'minutes', 'B' means 'hours' and 'C' means 'days or longer'.

If you have further queries about the complementary therapies listed, contact the Natural Medicine Society (see appendix 4). If you have further queries about the orthodox therapies, your doctor should be able to advise you.

TREATMENT	HOW DO YOU GET IT?	WILL IT HELP?	WILL IT HURT?	WILL IT HARM?	COST	TIME
Analgesics	Chemist Doctor	Maybe – certainly in the relief of mild pain	No	Only if you fail to follow directions	A/B	A
Anti-inflammatory drugs	Doctor	Maybe – certainly in the relief of mild pain	No	Yes if you fail to follow direct	A/B	A
Anti-depressants	Doctor	Maybe – but should be viewed with caution	No	Yes if you fail to follow directions	A/B	A
Narcotic drugs	Doctor	Maybe – but these are very strong	No	Yes if you become addicted	C	A

TREATMENT	HOW DO YOU GET IT?	WILL IT HELP?	WILL IT HURT?	WILL IT HARM?	COST	TIME
Tranquillisers	Doctor	Maybe – but should be viewed with caution	No	Yes if you fail to follow directives	A/B	A
Bedrest	Own steam	Maybe	No	No	Free	C
Heat/Cold	Own steam Physiotherapist	Maybe	Yes if you overdo it and burn yourself or get frostbite	No	Free or A	B
Electrical treatments	Physiotherapist	Maybe	Yes if you overdo it	No	A/B	B
Collars and corsets	Own steam Doctor	Maybe	No	No	A/B	C

Treatment	Physiotherapist				A/B	B
Traction		Maybe – but out of fashion at present	Rarely	No	A/B	B
Auto suspension	Own steam Doctor	Maybe – but probably no better than ordinary traction	No	Possibly if you suffer from giddiness	A/B	B
Massage and manipulation	Osteopaths Chiropractors Some doctors Some physiotherapists	Maybe – we practise manipulation among other things	No – unless the clinician is very rough	Possibly, especially if you suffer from giddiness	B/C	B/C

TREATMENT	HOW DO YOU GET IT?	WILL IT HELP?	WILL IT HURT?	WILL IT HARM?	COST	TIME
Local anaesthetic injections	Doctor	Maybe	Any injection hurts a little	Not if you are in good hands	A/B	A
Steroid injections	Doctor	Maybe	Any injection hurts a little	Not if you are in good hands	A/B	A
Epidural injections	Doctor	Maybe	Any injection hurts a little	Not if you are in good hands	A/B	A
TENS	Doctor Physiotherapist Own steam	Maybe	Rarely	Not if you are in good hands	A/B	A/B

					A/B	A/B
Acupuncture Acupressure	Doctor Acupuncturist Self	Maybe Maybe	Maybe No	Not if you are in good hands	Free	B
Rhizolysis and rhizotomy	Surgeon	Maybe	Yes	Not if you are in good hands	B	B
Nerve root surgery	Surgeon	Often	Yes	Rarely	C	C
Disc surgery	Surgeon	Often	Yes	Rarely	C	C
Chemonucleolysis	Surgeon	Maybe	Yes	Maybe	C	C
Sclerosant therapy	Doctor	Maybe	Yes	No	B	B
Hypnosis	Hypnotherapist – check reputable	Maybe	No	Maybe – if hypnotherapist not reputable	B	B

TREATMENT	HOW DO YOU GET IT?	WILL IT HELP?	WILL IT HURT?	WILL IT HARM?	COST	TIME
Biofeedback and relaxation response	Doctor	Maybe	No	No	B	B
Behavioural and cognitive behaviour therapies	Doctor	Often	No	No	A/B	C
Psychotherapy and counselling	Psychotherapist Counsellor	Maybe	No	No	B	B/C
Exercise	Self	Maybe	Not unless you overdo it	Not unless you overdo it	Free	C

CONCLUSION If you try any of these treatments and it fails to work, change it! Keep an open mind about treatments. Do not trust a dogmatic clinician.

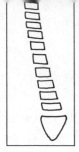

CHAPTER 9

People who may help

In this chapter we look at a number of different groups of people who could treat your back. As it is *your* back it is only reasonable that you should want to know the answers to some questions. In each case we try to answer these questions.

- How do you find your chosen clinician?
- What sort of person will your chosen clinician be?
- What will your chosen clinician do?
- Will your chosen clinician hurt you?
- What risks do you run?

Many of the professions listed below have umbrella organisations to which any reputable practitioner will belong. Addresses of these umbrella organisations are given in appendix 4. The umbrella organisations will be able to advise you about the relevant complementary therapist in your area; your doctor will advise you about other orthodox practitioners you may see.

Acupuncturists

How do you get an acupuncturist? In almost every case you make an appointment on the recommendation of someone who has found acupuncture helpful.

What sort of person will an acupuncturist be? Their training may be quite extensive and there are an increasing number of doctors practising acupuncture. However, there is nothing in law to stop anyone from buying a few needles and setting up in practice as an acupuncturist. There is no generally accepted qualification and standards vary enormously, so do be careful when choosing an acupuncturist.

What will they do? They will insert fine needles into various parts of your body, sometimes surprisingly far away from your pain. They may leave them in for some time, occasionally giving them a twiddle. Sometimes they may pass an electric current through the needles. There is also a form of acupuncture, called *electro-acupuncture*, in which no needles are used, but a current is passed through a blunt probe (electrode), placed lightly on your skin.

Will they hurt you? They should not; if they do, make sure you tell them.

What risks do you run? None, except for the possibility of infection from an unsterile needle. This is very rare, though it is something you should bear in mind in view of AIDS.

Alexander Technique Teachers

How do you get to a teacher? Your doctor may recommend one or you can apply directly to the Society of Teachers of the Alexander Technique (STAT) for a list of teachers (see appendix 4).

What sort of person will they be? Teachers who have undertaken a three-year training and try to help you help yourself.

What will they do? Pupils are taught by hand contact and verbal instructions how to avoid preparatory tightening before movement and eliminate the harmful habits which may often cause pain.

Will they hurt you? No, nothing in the Alexander Technique is hurtful.

What risks do you run? Because of the nature of the Technique and the training of the teachers there are no risks.

Back specialists

How do you get a back specialist? By referral by your family doctor.

What sort of person will a back specialist be? First they will be a doctor. If they are a *rheumatologist* or an *orthopaedic surgeon*, they will have had a specialist training after qualifying in medicine. But back problems are so common, disabling and difficult to deal with, that many other doctors from different branches of medicine try to deal with them, and, later, become specialists in this field. There are almost as many approaches to back problems within the medical profession as there are outside it, and really the back specialist may be one of a number of doctors from widely differing backgrounds. Who you see will depend on the judgement of your GP. What all specialists have in common is a medical qualification and an interest in your back.

What will they do? They will take a history and examine you. They may ask for laboratory tests, if they think it necessary. How they treat you will depend upon their background and particular interests – injections, manipulation, drugs, acupuncture or hypnosis are all treatments they may consider. Only a trained surgeon will operate on your back.

Will they hurt you? This depends upon what they do. Some treatments are bound to hurt a bit, for example injections.

What risks do you run? Because their qualifications follow a thorough training, the risk of damage to your back are as small as for other well-qualified groups.

Bone-setters

How do you get a bone-setter? In country areas you can find bone-setters by word of mouth; it is your decision to use one, your doctor will not recommend a bone-setter. Bone-setters are rare in urban areas. Bone-setters have no umbrella organisation.

What sort of person will a bone-setter be? They will probably have had no formal training or qualification. They will probably have learned their skill from their father or another member of their family.

What will they do? They will manipulate you. There is a good chance of their helping you.

Will they hurt you? They should not, but if they do, let them know straight away. If they say it is bound to hurt, go home and think of someone else to go to.

What risks do you run? We have discussed the dangers of manipulation already. The rare disasters may be avoided *only* if the bone-setter knows how your body works and what can go wrong with it. This needs proper training.

Chiropractors

How do you get to a chiropractor? This is usually something you determine on a personal recommendation. In this country it is still rare for your doctor to send you to a chiropractor, although this attitude is changing. In the United States, and in parts of Europe, chiropractors are widely used and widely respected. The British Chiropractic Association will be able to recommend a practitioner in your area.

What sort of person will a chiropractor be? In this country chiropractors should be formally trained, belonging to a professional body such as the British

Chiropractic Association, but there are some without formal training. They concern themselves mostly with bone and joint problems and you may find chiropractic treatments helpful with back pain.

What will they do? In trying to make a diagnosis, they will usually arrange for you to be X-rayed. On the evidence we can find, X-rays are really needed for diagnoses in only a very small proportion of back problems and the information they provide is very limited. So X-rays seem to us to be usually an unnecessary expense. The treatment the chiropractor will give you is in general limited to massage and manipulation. They may speak of *subluxation* (when part of a joint has slipped) and *adjustment* (putting something back into place). They will differ from the osteopath by usually using more force in what they do.

Will they hurt you? They may. Some chiropractors believe in using very considerable force, and this may hurt you.

What risks do you run? The law in this country allows anybody to offer you treatment of almost any kind. So you must choose very carefully to whom you go. We stress again that you must check that your chosen chiropractor is properly trained.

GPs

How do you get to them? Almost all of you will be registered with an NHS doctor. We include GPs here for the sake of completeness, although many of you will be familiar with the information we now provide.

What sort of person will they be? They will be one of 30,000 in this country who will have trained in a teaching hospital. After qualifying they will, by law, have had to undergo further training to become a GP. About a quarter of their work in general practice will have to do with bones and joints, but unfortunately their training is woefully inadequate. As doctors, we are campaigning to have doctors' training with regard to back problems improved – and improved quickly.

What are they likely to do? Usually GPs will prescribe pain-killers, and sometimes other drugs. Your GP should have due regard to possible side-effects from drugs and be able to explain to *you* what any side-effects might be. Your GP may send you to bed. Nobody really knows how this helps. As staying in bed may not be as helpful as early mobilisation and may in itself become a bad habit for you, it is wise to look at other possibilities. Your GP may arrange an X-ray of your back. In many cases this will not help because most back pain originates in muscles and ligaments, which do not show up on X-ray. If you are in great pain, if your pain fails to get better, or if your GP makes a diagnosis of disease, he or she may send you to a consultant. What GPs are *not* likely to do is to use massage or manipulation, although about 400 out of 30,000 family doctors do recommend or offer these treatments. They are also unlikely to use hypnotherapy or acupuncture.

Will your GP hurt you? This depends upon which of the many treatments available they choose. Generally speaking, they will not hurt you. If the recommended treatment is likely to involve pain, your GP will warn you of this.

What risks do you run? Because of their training in general medicine, the risk of your doctor doing you a mischief is very small.

Herbalists

How do you get to a herbalist? A register of medical herbalists is available upon application to the Secretary of The National Institute of Medical Herbalists (see appendix 4 for the address and telephone number). Most herbalists advertise in Yellow Pages but the best way is always through personal recommendation. Look for MNIMH or FNIMH after the name.

What sort of person will they be? All Members of the National Institute of Medical Herbalists have undergone a four-year training.

What is a herbalist likely to do? The first consultation will last about one hour, during which past medical problems and family illnesses as well as the present trouble will be discussed. Any relevant psychological pressures will be taken into consideration when prescribing the herbal remedy. An examination of the back and possibly other joints will be carried out, if necessary. Dietary and exercise advice will be given, if required, and a herbal prescription is usually given right away.

Will they hurt you? No, but the medicine may taste unpleasant!

What risks do you run? None.

Homoeopaths

How do you get to them? The most common route is by recommendation. A less satisfactory method is to refer to Yellow Pages: look out for the initials RS Hom (Registered Member of the Society of Homoeopaths). Many health food shops and pharmacies carry details of local practitioners. The Society of Homoeopaths supplies a register of professional practitioners and the British Homoeopathic Association one of doctors with varying levels of homoeopathic training (for addresses and telephone numbers, see appendix 4).

What sort of person will they be? There are two major categories of homoeopathic practitioner: the first are those who have undergone a formal training at recognised colleges; the second are orthodox doctors who have undergone postgraduate training in homoeopathy.

What will they do? A homoeopath will need a detailed case history in order to decide on the most appropriate prescription. Information will be needed about current symptoms, past medical history, family medical history, overall level of health, and how the current problem may be affecting the patient emotionally. All of this detailed information is necessary in order to establish how ill-health is affecting the person as an individual, which is why common symptoms may be of less interest to a homoeopath. As well as dispensing the relevant homoeopathic prescription (usually in tablet form), many homoeopaths will give general advice on relaxation techniques or changes in lifestyle that may be helpful.

Will they hurt you? No.

What risks do you run? Homoeopathic treatment can provide a safe and effective option for those who are in pain. If a homoeopathic prescription is inaccurate, the most likely outcome is lack of response. Homoeopathy can be used in a supportive context to other therapies such as osteopathy or chiropractic.

Medical manipulators

How do you get to them? Bone-setters, chiropractors and osteopaths all offer forms of manipulation, but none of these is a *medical* manipulator, because none of them has a formal medical training. Your family doctor may be one of the few hundred who use manipulation as a method of treatment for your back. If they are not one of these few, then they may refer you to a colleague who does.

What will a medical manipulator do? Doctors, will, of course, be in a position to use other treatments, if manipulation does not help.

Will they hurt you? Medical manipulators should not hurt you. If they do, make sure you say so.

What risks do you run? Because of their training, there will be no more risks than for any doctor.

Neurosurgeons

For the purposes of this book, we can say a neurosurgeon differs little from an orthopaedic surgeon. There are at present about 50 neurosurgeons in this country. Their training is rigorous, and they offer treatments very similar to these offered by orthopaedic surgeons.

Orthopaedic surgeons

How do you get to them? You are sent by your family doctor.

What sort of person an orthopaedic surgeon be? They will be a doctor who specialises in the surgery of bones and joints who will have had at least eight years' training after graduating as a doctor. There are about 700 or 800 of them in this country.

What will they do? They will take a history and examine you, possibly ordering laboratory tests and almost certainly asking for X-rays. More often than not, they will do their best *not* to operate on your back. So do not think that being sent to an orthopaedic surgeon means that you are doomed to an operation! Your doctor will usually have sent you to them for investigation and/ or physiotherapy. They may use injections or manipulation. If they do decide on an operation, they will not do so lightly. They will be able to explain to you the pros and cons of surgery so that you can make an informed decision about whether you want to proceed with an operation.

Will they hurt you? They should not hurt you on examination but, if they decide on surgery you will have a certain amount of pain.

What risks do you run? All major surgery carries risks and therefore will not be lightly offered. Indeed, it will only be used if there are indications that other therapies have failed. Surgery has a 50 per cent success rate in relieving back pain.

Osteopaths

How do you get to them? Ask your GP, enquire at your local hospital or health centre, look in the Yellow Pages or Thomson Directory, ring Talking Pages, or contact the Osteopathic Information Service.

What sort of person will they be? The osteopathic profession now has statutory regulation meaning that, in future, all osteopaths will meet the same high standards of training and clinical practice, be covered by professional indemnity insurance, and adhere to a professional code of practice.

What will they do? An osteopath will take a very detailed case history. He/she will want to know about the present problem and the patient's previous medical history. The osteopath will examine not only the area which is painful but also other related parts of the body.

The procedure is very similar to a conventional medical examination and, when necessary, osteopaths will request X-rays as part of the diagnostic procedure.

Will they hurt you? Osteopathic treatment involves the use of predominantly gentle forms of manual treatment and most patients find treatment a relaxing and pleasant experience.

What risks do you run? None.

Pain clinics

How do you get there? Pain clinics are a marvellous inovation which we discuss further in the final chapter. For the moment it is enough to say that they are centres bringing together a range of specialists to advise patients on pain management. You are referred to a pain clinic either by your family doctor or by a consultant.

Who will you see there? Pain clinics aim to relieve the suffering of those with persistent pain, and help those with chronic pain to live as nearly normally as possible, at home and at work. They are usually run by a consultant anaesthetist, because these people already have a special interest in relieving pain and much experience of giving difficult injections. With the anaesthetist will be more doctors and also other professionals from different backgrounds, such as psychologists, counsellors and physiotherapists. As we have mentioned before, pain is dealt with by many medical specialities and it has both physical and mental components. The idea of the pain clinic is to bring together various clinicians and specialists so that they can all contribute to fighting your pain. If you attend a pain clinic there is a high chance you will be helped.

What will they do for you? Professionals working at pain clinics may use a variety of treatments, including injections, acupuncture and hypnosis. They will use any treatment that relieves your pain, providing it is safe. Pain clinics also run courses for professionals from different fields to educate them in managing pain. Those few whose pain they fail to cure will be taught how to live as fully as possible despite the pain.

Will they hurt you? While this depends upon what treatments are given to you, it is very unlikely that anything painful will be done to you in a pain clinic.

What risks do you run? There are so many treatments you may be offered in the pain clinic that some are bound to carry a limited risk. On the other hand, there is plenty of help available, if needed.

Physiotherapists

How do you get to them? Usually, you will have been to your GP, who will have sent you either straight to the physiotherapy department of your local hospital or, more likely, to a consultant neurosurgeon, consultant rheumatologist, or an orthopaedic surgeon. Any of these consultants may send you to a physiotherapist. A number of physiotherapists also practise privately, some in association with sports clubs. You may, of course, go directly to these, or on the recommendation of your sports coach.

What sort of person will a physiotherapist be? Physiotherapists have a four-year basic training. There are about 30,000 in this country; roughly half of them deal with bone, and joint rehabilitation. This means helping you to get back to normal activity after any disabling illness. The physiotherapist's position is changing; while in the past they took instructions from doctors, now they are more independent, because they often know more about pain problems than the doctors. It is likely they will see you more often and be in a better position to note your improvements than other clinicians. This is understood in many hospitals, where the physiotherapists may alter your treatment as they think fit. If the pain-killers your doctor gave you do not help, you are likely to end up with a physiotherapist.

What will a physiotherapist do? A physiotherapist may use a number of treatments, each with its advantages and its disadvantages. None of these treatments should hurt.

The main treatments used by physiotherapists are:

- Heat and cold – these are often helpful and are quite harmless, if properly used.
- Electrical treatments – for example, ultrasound, short-wave diathermy, and interferential therapy. The way these work is not fully understood, but they are often helpful and they are harmless, if used by properly trained staff.
- Traction – again, no one knows quite how this works, but it is often successful and does no harm.
- Massage – this is a good treatment and will often give you great comfort. It works in the same way as manipulation, although it generally takes much longer.
- Manipulation – a considerable number of physiotherapists in this country use manipulation of different types. You may find this helpful.
- Exercises – your physiotherapist may ask you to perform a number of simple exercises on a regular basis.

All these treatments were discussed at greater length in the last chapter.

What risks do you run? None, really, in the hands of a properly trained person. You also usually have the immediate back-up of the hospital, if you are not making satisfactory progress.

Psychiatrists

How do you get a psychiatrist? Usually you will have been referred by a consultant in another hospital department because your pain has not got better with other treatments. Being sent to a psychiatrist may upset you at first because you may assume that the psychiatrist thinks your problem is all in the mind, a suggestion which may make you angry, but it is now known, beyond any shadow of doubt, that chronic pain always has a psychological side to it, and may respond to psychological treatments. So, if other people have failed to help you, do try the psychiatrist. As we have already said, when your back pain is not getting better, another form of treatment is worth a try, provided it is safe.

What sort of person will he or she be? The psychiatrist will be a doctor who has spent many years of further training studying the mind after qualifying as a doctor.

What will they do? They will go into your history in great depth, looking for a psychological cause for your persistent pain. They will probably not examine or investigate you, as all this will have been done in another department. They will either prescribe drugs or some form of psychotherapy. This consists of trying to come to terms with the cause of your pain through discussion, and can be very helpful. A consultation with a psychiatrist carries no risk and will not hurt you.

Psychotherapists and Counsellors

Counsellors tend to address very specific, easily identifiable problems, whilst psychotherapists help you to understand less accessible, often unconscious, causes of emotional trauma. Both are concerned with the mental or emotional components of pain. Psychotherapists and counsellors may or may not be medically qualified. You may find yourself one or the other without referral from a doctor but they may both work in pain clinics and similar remarks apply to them as to psychiatrists.

Rheumatologists

How do you get to them? You are sent by your family doctor.

What sort of person will they be? Rheumatologists are doctors who specialise in rheumatic diseases. They do not do any operations. They will have had at least seven years' training after qualifying as a doctor. There are only about 250 rheumatologists in this country. In view of the scale of the problem this is far too few, and many NHS Area Health Authorities do not have a rheumatologist at all. Shortage of cash in the NHS has so far proved a real stumbling block to progress in this area, and this is unlikely to improve.

What will they do? The rheumatologist will take a history and examine you, and almost certainly order laboratory tests and X-rays. Depending on the results of these tests, they are likely to prescribe the drug they think best for you and/or some physiotherapy. They may give you an injection or even manipulate you, but they are not very likely to prescribe any other form of treatment.

Will they hurt you? This is unlikely, but if they do, you must tell them. You run no risks from a rheumatologist.

Sports coaches

How do you get to them? Most sports and fitness clubs have a coach or somebody who is supposed to give immediate help if an injury does occur.

What sort of person are sports coaches likely to be? Almost anybody may be a sports coach. They may be an osteopath or a physiotherapist, but are likely to have had little formal training.

What will they do? Sports coaches give an immediate response to injury; what they usually do will vary very widely, depending on circumstances and training.

Will they hurt you? They may. Make sure you tell them if they do.

What risks do you run? This raises an important point, because you really have very little choice if a sports coach is the only person available to help you after a sports injury and you need immediate help. But because of the variations in coaches' training you should be careful about accepting advice, particularly regarding exercise. Some of the exercises recommended may actually do you harm. Being a good coach does not necessarily mean being an expert on backs! Standardised training of sports coaches would be helpful.

Sports medicine specialists

How do you get to a sports medicine specialist? By referral through your family doctor.

What sort of person will he or she be? Usually they will be either an orthopaedic surgeon or a rheumatologist who has developed a particular interest in sports medicine. Some may be general practitioners.

What will they do? They will take a history and examine you and usually have X-rays taken. They may send you for physiotherapy, give you an injection or, occasionally, manipulate you.

Will they hurt you? They may. So say so! But because of their medical training risks are few.

CONCLUSION

There is a vast number of people you can turn to for help if you are a back pain sufferer. We have tried to describe the functions of some of these people, and to give you information you will need if you are to make informed choices about your clinician and treament and to participate fully in discussion once a treatment has been prescribed. If you are being looked after by someone from one of the groups we discuss but are making no progress, it is always worth asking what other help is available. You should keep an open mind, even if this sometimes puts you on a collision course with your clinician. If your clinician does not seem to be making any progress, change him or her! If your clinician does not keep an open mind, but is dogmatic in approach, change him or her! If a treatment is not working, demand that it be changed!

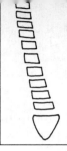

CHAPTER 10

Consultations – good and bad

We have tried to give you an overview both of possible treatments and the people who give them. We now offer suggestions as to how you can tell the good consultation from the bad, *whoever* you decide to approach for help. Our aim is partly to stop you being conned by unscrupulous people who might otherwise take advantage of your pain for financial gain, i.e. practitioners of all sorts. More generally, we want to help you make sure you get the right clinician, whatever their speciality. When comparing the good consultation and the bad consultation we consider six key indicators:

- The nature of the history taken.
- The nature of the examination given.
- How your problem and its treatment are explained to you.
- The treatment prescribed.
- Use of laboratory tests and X-rays.
- Cost.

THE GOOD CONSULTATION

History

Because of the enormous number of factors which can contribute to your pain, the person you consult needs to gain a full picture, not only of your present problem, but also of the sort of life you lead, your general health and your previous medical history. No one can do this properly in a hurry. We have already discussed the great difficulties which face clinicians in making an accurate diagnosis and at every follow-up visit your medical history will need to be thoroughly up-dated so that if no progress is being made, the treatment may be changed accordingly. You should feel confident that the person whose help you are seeking is prepared to spend time on your history and to seek clarification if anything is unclear. You should also feel free to ask questions of them.

Examination

Examination must be extensive and pains-taking; this means it will be time-consuming. Examination of your whole spine must be included in every case of back pain. This will lessen the confusion which arises if the physical signs are widespread. After every treatment the examination must be repeated. The person performing it must look for changes in the signs which were originally found. Apart from what you can tell him or her about your symptoms, this is the only way the examiner knows whether treatment is progressing and will allow them to decide on the wisest next step. Of course, the examination must also be repeated at every follow-up visit.

Explanation

Any consultation should include an explanation of what your clinician thinks is causing your pain and what they propose to do about it. It must also give you full answers to any questions you may have. Because of the difficulties in accurate diagnosis, the explanation may seem to you to be not as clear-cut as you might have wished or expected. In fact, in view of what we have already said about diagnosis, the therapist who appears rather hesistant may well know more than a colleague with a quick answer. So such a hesitant, thoughtful therapist may well be the safer person and is more likely to change your treatment if it is necessary. This will be to your advantage.

Treatment

The clinician who is prepared to change what they are doing if it is not succeeding knows more about your problem than the one who sticks to the same old treatment, whatever happens. After the prescription of pain-killers, manipulation is the most frequently used treatment for your back pain, so it is important for you to know that this should not hurt. You should make sure that any of the treatments you are offered is safe – ask if you are unsure of anything. If surgery is recommended, make sure your clinician spells out all the pros and cons and do not be afraid to continue asking questions until everything is clear in your mind. If you want a second opinion, ask for one.

Laboratory tests and X-rays

Tests and investigations, particularly X-rays, are seldom of help in making an accurate diagnosis. For example, the X-ray appearances of ageing in your spine are usually to be seen when you are little over 30 and become more prominent over the rest of your life, whether you have back pain, or not! Therefore, in a good consultation, a clear explanation must be given as to how the X-ray investigation and other laboratory tests may help in your case.

Cost

If you are paying for the treatment yourself it is important that your clinician is able to give you a scale of charges and to give you some indication of the total cost of your treatment. Be very wary of clinicians who cannot spell out your likely financial commitment; you might be in for a nasty surprise when it comes to paying the bills!

THE BAD CONSULTATION

History

The consultation seems rushed, your chosen clinician skates over details which you think are important and does not give you a chance to comment. Little or no history is taken. No proper history is sought at follow-up visits.

Examination

A sketchy and rapid examination is made, that does not include the whole of your back. No examination is made after treatment. No examination is made at follow-up visits.

Explanation

An over-confident and clear-cut diagnosis is given, based on little history and hurried examination. You should ask for an explanation of diagnosis and why the treatment being offered has been chosen.

Treatment

If the treatment hurts more than a very little, you should be on your guard. If the same treatment is given time after time, when you do not seem to be making real progress, it strongly suggests that this is not suitable for you. The therapist may be banging the drum for some very particular interpretation of your problem. If at the start you are recommended a long course of treatment, you should be very wary. This may be better business than therapy.

Laboratory tests and X-rays

When tests are suggested as a matter of course, you should be on the alert for the other signs of the bad consultation – again this may be better business than therapy.

Cost

Some practitioners may be very unwilling to discuss costs or to indicate the size of the final bill – beware!

To summarise the discussion of the good and the bad consultation we will just say that if you have any doubts at all that the people supposed to be helping you and the treatments they are offering are not doing you any good or are not in your best interests, then ask questions. If you are not given satisfactory answers then consider changing practitioners. If you choose to go to a complementary therapist, always use someone who is a member of the relevant umbrella organisation, if there is one. Addresses for these bodies can be found in appendix 4.

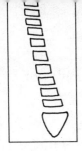

CHAPTER 11

Acute pain – self-help

IMMEDIATE ACTION

All pain has a beginning, runs its course and usually comes to an end. In *acute pain* the course is usually short. If you have a sudden and severely painful attack of back pain there is little you can do, except to lie down in the position which gives you least pain. At first, back pain can be quite frightening, but usually within hours it settles down enough to allow you to make some movements. The important thing is not to do anything which makes your pain worse, so rely on pain-killers and wait. There is no point in sending for your doctor at this stage, unless you find difficulty in controlling your bladder or bowels, or you develop pins and needles or numbness. If you do develop any of these symptoms at any time with back pain, you must get in touch with your doctor and let him know about it straight away.

You may find that either a hot water bottle or a cold compress helps at this stage, but if your pain is really severe for more than four or five hours, it is reasonable to send for your doctor, who may send you into hospital.

Staying in bed

If, as is most often the case, the agonising pain settles down enough to allow some movement, the best place for you is in bed. You must stay there. There has been much debate on the best kind of bed for bad backs. The simple answer is that the best bed for you is the one in which you are most comfortable, be it hard or soft. If you think your bed is too hard, then it is worth trying to find a softer one. On the other hand, if it seems too soft, you can either put a board under the mattress or put the mattress on the floor. You will probably have to get someone else to make these changes for you. But remember that the common advice to put a board under the mattress may not suit you. So do not stick with this idea, if you find it is of no help. Certainly do not be conned into spending a fortune on a so-called 'orthopaedic bed' – or on any item without trying it out first, and not just for a day. The National Back Pain Association has a list of suppliers who will let you try out beds and other items of back pain furniture before you buy.

You are bound to find difficulty in eating or drinking in bed. You may find it worthwhile trying a bent straw for drinking. It is sensible to eat and drink as little as possible in the early stages, so as to reduce the need for you to go to the toilet. Do not worry if you are a bit constipated, for this is quite normal in anyone confined to bed. When you do have to go, try to get to the bathroom rather than perching on a bed pan as this is generally less of a problem. In order to get out of bed when you are in pain, it is best to roll to the edge of the bed, bring your knees up and drop your feet over the side. Then sit up sideways and use a chair near the bed for support. You may find it more comfortable to crawl than trying to walk.

Pain relief

In the first two or three days, you should find some help through pain-killers. Use those you have found helpful in the past. A hot water bottle applied to that part which hurts most is often quite helpful, but remember that you need to keep it there for at least 20 minutes to do any good. If it is too hot on its own, wrap it in a towel. Some people find using an ice-pack more help. A satisfactory home-made ice-pack is a packet of frozen peas. It will mould itself into your shape and you can put it back in the fridge after use! If heat does not work, try cold and vice versa. Some find it most helpful to switch from heat to cold, perhaps alternating it several times.

Ointments, such as Algipan, can be helpful and are harmless. Applying the ointment involves gentle massage, which you may find brings comfort in itself. You can ask a member of your family to massage the painful part, but do tell them to stop if it hurts you. If you are interested in aromatherapy, it might be worth trying an aromatherapy massage.

AFTER THE THIRD DAY

If by the third day you are no better, then you will have to call in your family doctor. Before deciding what to do they will want to know whether there is anything seriously wrong with you and may order X-rays or laboratory tests to rule out, or in rare cases to confirm, the presence of disease. Your GP will almost certainly advise you to stay in bed, and may prescribe a stronger pain-killer. At this point you will probably need a medical certificate for your employer and your doctor should provide one. If your pain fails to settle down in the next week or two, your doctor will probably wish to send you to an orthopaedic surgeon, a rheumatologist, a neurosurgeon or a physiotherapist. By this time, you will probably have started thinking of trying other treatments, many of which we discussed in chapter 8. If your pain does last more than three days, you may begin to worry about its long-term effect on your life, we will discuss this issue in the next two chapters.

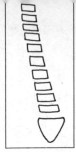

CHAPTER 12

Chronic pain – prevention

We talked about what you can do in an attack of *acute* back pain in chapter 11. Here we discuss your role in self-help in *chronic* back pain and its prevention. *Chronic* pain is pain which takes a long time to run its course. We deal with chronic pain prevention at home and in the garden, at work and when travelling.

Because an accurate diagnosis of back pain is rarely possible, do not persist with the advice we give if it is not helping you, and certainly not if it is causing you pain. As the cause of your pain is almost always unknown, no one can be sure of how to prevent it. Nevertheless, the advice we give should be helpful, but if in your particular case you find it actually brings on the pain, we repeat that you must stop whatever it is you are doing. If any activity causes you pain you should try to analyse for yourself what is going wrong; a solution might be obvious.

AT HOME, IN THE GARAGE AND IN THE GARDEN

Hoovering

This can cause back problems because you are usually stooping a bit and pulling or pushing a heavy, vibrating machine; all this puts pressure on your spine. You can reduce the effects by choosing a machine which allows you to stand up straight; this means either one with a long enough handle or one with a flexible suction hose. In the first instance you are still doing as much pulling and pushing, but at a more suitable height. In the second you are having to move the machine itself only from time to time. If you still get pain on hoovering plan to do the job in several short stints, or if you can afford it, get help with your housework. This applies to every job which causes you back pain, both in coping with it and in trying to avoid it.

Washing the floor

It is best to remain standing when cleaning the floor so you need a long-handled mop or squeegee. You can also avoid putting a strain on your back by doing the cleaning on hands and knees, provided you keep your back hollowed, i.e. you maintain your *lumbar lordosis*. This involves sticking your bottom out – advice which goes for many activities which risk causing back pain! It may not be very elegant but it may save you a great deal of trouble! Remember also that carrying two half buckets of water is better than one full one.

Hanging curtains – or taking them down

Dealing with curtains often puts a strain on your neck and upper back, as you are in an awkward position for quite a time and reaching up to take what may be a considerable weight. There are two things which may help. The first is to stand on something, so that you are working at a more comfortable level, but make sure what you stand on is safe. The second is to take several bites at the cherry. Hang or take down one pair of curtains, then do something else for a while before returning for another session.

Hanging out the washing

This presents just the same problems as hanging curtains, maybe made worse by the extra weight of water in the wet clothes. So, either stand on something of a suitable height, or bring the line down to the level at which you find it most comfortable to work. Since hanging out the washing is such a frequent activity, it is worth persisting until you have a system that is right for you. Perhaps an adjustable-height drying rack might be the answer, if you have the room for it.

Ironing

Too often you stoop over too low an ironing board for too long at a time. Of course, you may choose to do the ironing sitting down, in which case you need the board pretty low, but if you iron standing up you must have the board high enough so that you stand up straight. Whichever position you choose, you will find it less of a strain on your back if the board is at about the level of your navel.

Shopping

You should carry your shopping divided equally between your two hands. You may find a lightweight trolley helpful. Be careful about loading and unloading the car boot with heavy shopping. When doing this keep your back straight and lift from the knees and try not to twist your body as you lift or put down the bags.

At the sink

For the back pain sufferer, the sink is one of the most important items of kitchen equipment, because it is here that you spend many hours preparing vegetables, washing up, etc., and this means standing in one position for long periods. Unfortunately, most kitchen designers seem to forget that the working height of your sink is its bottom, which means that you are stooping for much of your sink time. Also, most sinks are set some distance from the front edge of the working surface and as there

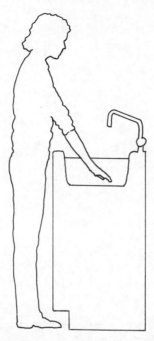

is seldom enough room to get your feet well under the sink, you have to lean forwards all the time. If you have a back problem, you have to consider all these points. If you cannot change the design of your kitchen, all you can do is to avoid working at your sink for any long periods or do the washing up in a bowl on the draining board.

Other kitchen working surfaces

Ideally these should be as near your waist level as possible and you should be able to get your feet close enough to or under the working surface to let your tummy rest against its edge. It is a mistake to plan a kitchen with all the work surfaces at the same height as different tasks and different height people need different height surfaces. If possible, vary the height of the surfaces by using different widths of plinth at the base of the units. High shelves and cupboards have the same

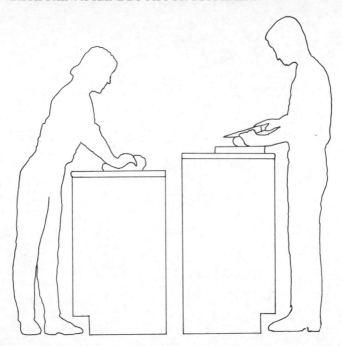

snags as hanging curtains and need the same answers. And, of course, the height of your oven should not make you stoop or reach.

Sitting in comfort

The easy chair and the sofa are often too soft to give your back the support it needs, are too low to get in and out of in safety and comfort, and give little or no support to your neck. If you get pain sitting in a soft, low chair, a sensible alternative is to use a hard, high chair, giving good support. Try not to sit with a rounded back, as this may lead to symptoms.

If you are watching television, it is worth placing your chair directly in front of the set, unless this causes family feuds. If you are reading, knitting or sewing for long periods, remember that you may give yourself a neck problem – so be ready to do something else if it starts to hurt and do not press on regardless.

If you do a lot of reading, you may find it helpful to use a book stand but do not invest in one until you have found out whether or not it helps. Borrow one if you can. The same advice applies to buying one of the many special chairs designed for the back sufferer. These can be very helpful but the only way you can find out is by trial and error. Do not spend a fortune, unless you know it is worth it for you. If you cannot find a chair which supports your back, you may find that a *lumbar roll*, or a rolling pin placed in the small of your back may help you.

These notes on sitting also apply to the work situation.

Shaving, washing your face, or making-up

Surprisingly, all three of these everyday activities are often the cause of back pain, sometimes severe. One reason, of course, may be that you are stooping over the basin for quite a long time. So, even in doing something which seems quite harmless, you may have to think about the position of your back. Your bathroom motto might well be, 'the straighter the safer'. And you may need to put your mirror higher on the wall or change its position so you do not have to twist to look into it.

Cleaning the bath

This can cause pain when stooping or reaching. Try getting into the bath to kneel or squat, so that everything is within easy reach. Kneeling on the floor beside the bath does not get rid of your having to reach to clean the other side. Incidentally, for back sufferers it is always best to have a bath with hand-holds, to help getting in and out of the bath.

Bed-making

Bed-making involves stooping and reaching, and both may be painful. The first thing you can do to reduce the risk is to kneel down when making the bed. You may find the use of a duvet a great help, as it means you do not have to lift and tuck in the bedclothes. Perhaps a higher bed would make life easier for you, both in bed-making and in getting in and out of bed. The bed is probably the most important piece of furniture in your life, for you are likely to spend something like 25 years lying in it. The many claims that this bed or that is best for your back cannot all be true and there are two things which make your choice difficult. First we are all different, and second there are so many possible causes for your back pain that they could not all be helped by one bed. The only way to find out which bed is best for you is by trial and error. It is not really enough just to lie down on one in the shop. You must try lying in different positions, preferably over a month or so. The moral of this must be that you should not spend a lot of money on a bed which is unlikely to be of help to you. When away from home you may find sleeping in a strange bed painful. If you are normally most comfortable on a firm bed, you could take a portable bedboard with you when travelling.

Back pain and sex

Back problems may affect your sex life, by causing pain to you or your partner if you have to ask him or her to adopt unusual positions to accommodate your problem. The key to a happy sex life for back pain sufferers and their partners is to experiment with different positions, so that if either of you is uncomfortable in one position, you can try another. If back pain is causing real problems in your sex life and this is making you or your partner miserable, ask your chosen clinician for advice.

Decorating

The two main problems which arise here are skirtings and ceilings. Skirtings may be best dealt with on your hands and knees, with your back hollowed. Ceilings can be a problem, particularly if you try to rush them. Dashing at the job too hard and for too long at one go whilst working with your head in an awkward position is a recipe for disaster. It pays to split the job into easy stages, even if it is not very popular with the family. Remember that long-handled rollers may help. Best of all, give up trying to do the decorating yourself and get someone in to do it for you, if you can afford this solution.

Moving furniture

This is best avoided! If you have to move furniture, empty cupboards and remove drawers before moving the carcase. You may find a length of strong material, such as upholsterers' webbing, useful as a sling under the legs of the piece to be moved and across your shoulders. If you do have to move heavy furniture, take enough time to plan it. The best solution is to leave moving furniture to other people.

In the garage

Inspecting the innards of your car means you will probably spend a long time stooping and reaching. Remember to change your activity as soon as you feel discomfort. If you have a back problem already, take particular care getting underneath the car and then standing up again. Again, the best solution might be to pay a mechanic to work on your car, if you can afford it.

In the garden

The jobs you have to do in the garden are often heavy.
Some involve stooping and lifting, which may be a cause
of painful episodes, and some may need machinery
which may be heavy and awkward to use. If you can
afford it, it might be best to hire a gardener to do your
heavy work. If you do not want to rely on someone else,
then follow the advice given now:

DIGGING

If digging hurts, you can try to reduce this in several
ways. You can use a spade with a long handle, which
means you can keep your back hollow and your bottom
sticking out. A larger handle gives you greater leverage.
You might also try one of a number of special spades
which are said to be easier to use – keep an eye out in
gardening catalogues for details of these. You must train
yourself to take a smaller amount of soil on each
spadeful not trying to get as much as possible on to your
spade each time. Lastly, as with any heavy work in the
garden or elsewhere, do not go on and on but take
planned breaks. The same advice applies to using a
garden fork.

HOEING

When using a long-handled hoe, whether a chopping or
pushing type, you may find it helps to keep your back
hollowed. However, it is more important to change jobs
frequently. With a short-handled hoe, you might
consider kneeling down.

WEEDING

As far as your back is concerned, weeding is a similar
activity to short-handled hoeing. You may find a
cushioned mat quite a comfort but the most important
thing is not to get carried away and go on too long.

LAWNMOWING

The dangers here are in stooping to start the machine, humping a heavy mower around corners, disposing of the grass-mowings and the basic height of the lawnmower handles. You may need to change the length of the starting cord, so that you can pull it from handle height, instead of having to bend down. Choose the lightest machine you can find; electric ones are usually lighter and do not need starting. Even if it seems very small for your lawn, it is better to take more runs with a small machine than to give yourself back pain by using a larger model. Handles vary in height, and if they are adjustable see that they are set at the height that suits you best. With regard to the disposal of mowings, it is far better to empty your grass box more often than to overload it – and your back! The same applies to using the wheelbarrow.

WHEELBARROWING

Very low handles make you bend down to pick them up. Do not try to wheel an overloaded barrow – extra journeys are better than pain. Whether you push or pull the barrow, carefully balance the weight and avoid twisting.

AT WORK

As work situations vary so much we will look at several different types and try to draw some general conclusions, so while you may not find exactly your job described you should nevertheless be able to find general principles which will help you prevent chronic pain arising from your work.

Office work

As an office worker, you are likely to be sitting for much of the day and if you stay in one position for a long time, this may produce back pain. If pain does develop, you should have a change of activity and try to move around or to take a walk. If you are hunched over papers all day it might be a good idea to try some neck stretching exercises in your lunch hour.

Office furniture has a vital role to play. You should refer back to the section on seating, as similar remarks about chairs apply to the work environment. Since we are all of different shapes and sizes, the arrangement of your desk and chair must be an individual matter and it is really for you to work out for yourself what is best for you. If you have a very long back and you cannot alter the height of your desk, you may need to put your seat lower. If you are short, you may need to raise the seat. If you are really worried about your back, it might be worth trying to persuade the personnel department to buy you some new furniture. You may find it helpful if your chair is designed with a curved back to support

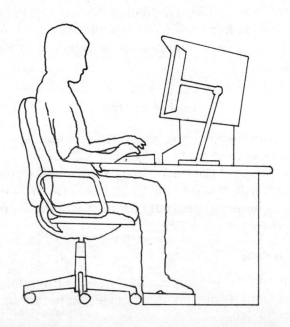

your spine and is adjustable, so your feet rest flat on the floor and your legs are flat against the seat.

If you are a typist, remember that you may be at particular risk, because you are likely to keep the same position for too long. You may also run into trouble if you are a VDU operator; changing the position of the machine may be helpful. Screens should be adjusted, so that your head is held straight when you are working. Eyes as well as backs are at risk for VDU operators.

It is now known that a telephonist may be at more risk than almost any other office worker, because the strain of lifting a telephone directory at arm's length causes a considerable rise of pressure inside the intervertebral discs. To avoid this telephonists must pull the directory near to their bodies before lifting it. Holding a telephone at an angle also influences back health. If your job involves using the telephone all the time, ask your boss to supply you with a hands-free headset, like those used by telephonists.

Heavy industry

You may be surprised to learn that, if you are in heavy industry, you will *not* develop back pain more often than anybody else. However, if you have a back problem and work in heavy industry, it is likely to be worse and to keep you from work longer. If problems develop, talk to your personnel officer, as well as to your clinician.

Assembly-line work

If you work on an assembly-line you are rather more likely than others to develop back pain, although *exactly* why is not quite clear. Over the past twenty-five years a great deal of research has been done, looking at working conditions, bench heights, etc., trying to relate these to sickness absence, but very little has resulted from all this

research. Again, if problems develop, talk to your
personnel department as well as to the doctors.

Nursing

You might think that, as they are likely to have to lift
heavy patients, nurses would have more back trouble
than, say, school teachers. This is just not so, although
nurses may suffer back pain at a younger age than
others. Nurses are taught to use their backs sensibly, to
lift from their knees, to hollow their backs when
standing at sinks and not to attempt too much in one go.

Farm work

There is no clear evidence as to whether farm work has
an adverse effect on the back, or not. It may be
reasonable to suggest that the farm worker of 50 years
ago kept physically fit all the year round, whereas today
his grandson sits on a bumpy tractor much of his time,
and that this leads to bad backs, but this view is only an
opinion.

Construction work

This is very variable and may involve heavy lifting and
carrying strains. If you are a bricklayer, you will know
that two-thirds of your work is too high or too low for
comfort, and mixing cement by hand is certainly tough
on your back. If you are a plumber or electrician, much
of your work will be in awkward positions. All sorts of
roofing involves hard physical work. Some serious back
injuries result from falling off ladders.

Lorry drivers

If you drive a lorry, you are likely to be troubled by the
vibration and by heavy steering and frequent gear
changing. If these things cause you pain, pull into a

layby, get out of the cab and walk about for a minute or two. If your job involves you in loading and unloading, then you have a whole new set of problems to think about. We give advice on lifting at the end of this chapter.

TRAVEL

Public transport

You may find that you spend much time standing at bus stops or on railway platforms. If you can plan your travel to avoid the rush hour, you may save yourself a lot of trouble. If you have a long wait, walk up and down, even if it means losing your place in the bus queue. Even if you do get a seat on a bus or a train, you may find the vibration uncomfortable, if so, see if things improve if you stand instead. But if you give up your seat or cannot get one, you may find strap-hanging and jostling with fellow passengers are also sources of pain. There is nothing you can do about this, except avoid busy periods. If it is feasible, take a taxi whenever you can.

Cars

If you drive at all, you are twice as likely to get disc trouble as if you do not. If you drive every day, you are three times as likely to be troubled in this way – a sobering thought!

While driving you are sitting in one position for a long time. To minimise the risks of developing back pain, try to avoid protruding the head and neck forwards, especially in poor visibility, and a lumbar roll in the small of your back may be helpful. If you develop back pain, stop and walk about for a while – do not press on. Much has been written about the design of car seats. The ideal angle of the car seat and the height of the head support are what you find best suit you. Because of this, and because we are all different, there can be no such thing as the ideal seat, and you should bear this in mind when buying a car. It might be worth investing in a beaded seat cover as some people find these a help. The best positions for your steering wheel and for your wing mirrors are the ones you find most comfortable. You may find that power steering and/or an automatic gearbox help you, so bear this in mind if you are test-driving new cars. Although seat belts prevent you from being catapulted through the windscreen, the price you pay for this crash protection may be an increased severity of whiplash injury to your neck, if you do have a crash. This is because your body is held back, while your head has no support. Getting in and out of the car may hurt. When getting in, try sitting on the seat first, before swinging your legs in. When getting out swing your legs out before getting out of the car. One more risk to your back can be in loading and unloading the boot. It may help you to keep your back straight and bend your knees. It may also be helpful to lift anything in or out of the boot straight, and to move your feet, rather than to twist round.

Air travel

Take as little hand luggage as you can and divide it equally between both hands. Struggling with baggage trolleys is a source of back pain at times, so hire a porter, if you can. Plan as carefully as possible to reduce the time you stand about in airports; if you do have a long wait, walk around. Seats in aircraft can cause back pain, and you may have to sit for a very long time. It is, therefore, well worth your while trying to find a gangway seat, because you can then more easily get up and walk about, if you need to. You can now buy inflatable neck rests in most airports and it might be worth buying one for the flight.

Cycling

Although cycling is an excellent form of exercise for improving your heart and lung capacity and strengthening your legs, take it easy at first, and build up the amount you do gradually.

The harder you push on a pedal, the harder you have to pull on the handlebars. So cycling is really a form of lifting. As you are pushing with one foot at a time and pulling with both hands, it is also a form of twisting, so you may be at risk, if you are pedalling hard. If cycling causes back pain, change to a lower gear. You may need to raise your handlebars, too. And do not be too proud – you may find it better to get off and walk up the worst of the hills.

Walking

You may find this painful but on the other hand you may find it helps. If it hurts, you must either stop or slow down. This applies to walking on the flat, up hills and up steps or stairs.

GOLDEN RULES FOR LIFTING

You may wonder why we have not given a mass of detailed advice – especially about lifting and carrying. We feel that most proferred advice suffers from the same problem we have mentioned elsewhere – that nobody really knows. So it is left very much to you to work out your own salvation. However, there are a few golden rules which do apply to all lifting. They are:

- Plan the lift. Do you need help?
- Stand close to the object you are about to lift.
- Gain a good grip.
- Secure your foothold.

- Bend your knees.
- Ensure your back is straight.
- Lift without jerking.
- Once the object is lifted, move your feet to put the object down. Do not twist or stoop.

CONCLUSION

The advice we give in this chapter *may* be helpful to you in handling your pain and preventing further attacks. However, as has been said, no single cause has ever been identified applicable to back pain in general. This may sound pretty depressing, but it need not be so, for if nobody knows, nobody can tell you you are silly to try something! All sorts of contradictory advice is given by all sorts of different people; this is not only very confusing for you, but you may find your whole life ruled by a set of beliefs mistakenly held by one person or another. There is no need for you to have your life so ruled. It is really very simple: if it hurts, do not do it. Do anything and everything that does not hurt. What suits you matters more than what you may be told. Back pain is a complicated business, and every individual's problems, ideas and situation vary. If you realise this and know that much advice is based on no more than unproved ideas, you can be your own best help.

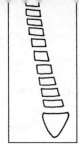

CHAPTER 13

Pain clinics

One of the ideas that has emerged over the past few years, and is widely recognised in pain clinics throughout the world, is that of the *chronic pain state*. This describes the unhappy situation in which pain, despite the best endeavours of various clinical advisers, cannot be cured. The chronic back pain sufferer may be one among many other sufferers in this state.

This creates a situation for both doctor and patient which has only recently received the attention it deserves. One of the features of Western medicine is that it tends to be geared to fairly short and intensive consultations, aimed at solving particular problems. If, however, a problem becomes chronic, as it can in pain of all sorts, then the situation requires longer interviews in which the details are dealt with in greater depth.

This is very important, because those of you with chronic back pain, unlike those suffering chronic conditions such as diabetes, heart disease or high blood pressure, usually do not have a clear-cut diagnosis and may not understand what is going on. This is because you may have seen many clinicians and have been given different opinions and explanations, and you are therefore confused.

You may have been told that nothing can be done for you, and that you must learn to live with your pain. Working with the National Back Pain Association, one often learns of members who have had a couple of treatments and an X-ray and been told that that is it, and that they have now got to put up with their pain; they are back pain rejects. But it is just not true that you have to put up with pain, and this chapter will make that point strongly. There are many factors, psychological and physiological, that determine whether you feel pain, or not. If you are aware of this, there is much more chance of your being helped and of your helping yourself.

Never accept you are a back pain reject

Never accept you are a back pain reject

Never accept you are a back pain reject

Never accept you are a back pain reject

As a back pain sufferer, you may develop a sense of helplessness, which in turn causes increasing anxiety and depression. You may feel that you have been abandoned. But this is quite wrong, for there is much that may be done.

A doctor who meets a patient with chronic pain, is probably meeting somebody who distrusts clinicians because of their past experiences. The sufferer may not understand their pain, and be confused, having goals as to what can be achieved in the chronic pain situation which are often very different from those of the doctor. This mis-match of expectation between doctor and patient can lead to all sorts of problems.

The perspective on your problem you and your doctor have may be different. Let us explain what this means. When you have pain, be it chronic or acute, you quite naturally hope that someone will get rid of it for you. But in the chronic pain state many treatments may have been tried and have failed. As we have said, there is nothing wrong in your seeking further help, provided that it is safe. But you should do so cautiously, because if you place too much hope in a new treatment and it fails yet again, the disappointment may add further to your troubles. However, your clinician may not only think that nothing can get rid of your pain and you must live with it, but may actively resist the idea of your trying to get help elsewhere; be firm and insist that this is what you want to do. You will not find this sort of mismatch between your views and those of clinicians at a pain clinic – this is just one of the positive factors which make pain clinics so helpful to patients.

THE PAIN PSYCHOLOGIST

The pain psychologist is a key member of the team at the pain clinic. He or she is not trying to abolish your pain; he or she is trying to reduce and even abolish the disability that chronic pain has brought to your life. The pain psychologist's approach may or may not result in reducing the frequency or intensity of your pain, but it should increase your activities and thereby improve the quality of your life. If it also reduces your pain, this is a bonus. First the psychologist explores your understanding of your problem, in order to identify misunderstandings and to correct them. You are then taught about the way you *think* (cognition), the way you *feel* (affect), and how you *behave* (the things you do in response to your pain). All of these interact the whole time (see chapter 5). All these factors influence each other in a way that may be harmful; your problems may persist and may even get worse. On the other hand, if you are aware of all three of these elements, you can positively improve your situation.

TAKING CONTROL OF YOUR LIFE

Clinicians at the pain clinic will encourage you to plan your own life and take charge of your situation. Many treatments involve your keeping a diary, so that you may understand what is happening to you. You are then encouraged to aim at reasonable goals of activity. It is important not to aim too high because, if you fail due to your pain, you will be more depressed and inclined to give up. If your goals are set at realistic levels, you can progressively do more and more each day. The amount of pain-killers you take is also of great importance. In many treatment programmes it has been found that the more pain-killers you take, the worse off you become. So the first item of business in most pain clinics is to cut down on these drugs. In contrast, you are encouraged to be more positive. For example, as already discussed, the more exercises you do, the fewer pain complaints you make and the less attention you pay to your pain. In other words, you are distracted by the things you actually do, rather than brooding over your situation. You are taught the skills of relaxation and controlled breathing. These and other similar techniques aim to give you something you can do yourself, if you feel your pain coming on. You feel less helpless when you have something you can do to control your pain. This is not only useful but helps your morale. Morale is a key factor for any chronic pain sufferer – if you feel miserable you are NOT being feeble, misery is a perfectly understandable reaction to pain.

Using the techniques taught at the pain clinic will give you an understanding of your problem and a repertoire of responses and practical hints to help you to lose your sense of helplessness and gain control. In doing this you increase what you can do and are able to live a fuller and more active life.

Your family

Your family may feel as helpless, as ignorant and, at times, as desperate as you. They may not understand your problem, they may feel defeated by it, and have to stand by not knowing how they can help you. But families are welcome at pain clinics, and if you give them the explanations we have given to you, they will understand the aims of your treatment and can play a part in helping you. Usually the pain clinic will insist your family be involved in treatment programmes and may help you to achieve your goals by encouraging you and trying to prevent you from slipping into bad habits. You and your family should be considered as a single unit, working together towards your recovery. Although they will not be brought into the pain clinic's network, it is best if you explain your treatment to friends and employers so that they can help too.

What these pain clinic programmes are trying to do is to give you an understanding of your problem and advice as to how you can improve your everyday life. The person at the centre of all this who has the most control over it is *you*. All your advisers, however distinguished they may be, are there only to give you advice. The key person is *you*. After all the advice you receive the heart of the matter lies in your realising that you are not helpless, defeated and rejected. With the right help and with the right attitude, you can do much for yourself. Maybe you cannot banish your pain, but you can do a very great deal to stop your pain banishing you and your family to a dreary existence.

Never accept you are a back pain reject

Never accept you are a back pain reject

Never accept you are a back pain reject

Never accept you are a back pain reject

CONCLUSION

You may say all these attitudes to pain management sound very fine, but what are the results? In fact they are extremely good, as some of the best research shows. One researcher ran a programme of treatment along the lines outlined here which showed significant improvement in a group of 36 patients over a period of nearly 2 years. This was confirmed by others, who reported that if back pain sufferers underwent a programme of 6–8 weeks involving the things we have discussed, then a follow-up period of 1–8 years, 20 out of 26 patients originally unemployed because of their pain were leading lives that were essentially normal from the point of view of function and employment. You have to admit that these are pretty good results.

CHAPTER 14

Conclusions

In the introduction, we described the present lack of back pain training for medical students and in general practice. We then set out to provide you with information about the various people who are available to help you. We also offered you a realistic picture of your own problems and what the many terms you hear actually mean. We hope to have achieved this, and in so doing to have provided you with a guide by which you can make up your own mind about what is best for you. If we have given you a clear enough picture of the realities you should feel more secure when faced with the sometimes fanciful ideas and advice you may receive, from whatever quarter.

We have also emphasised that in the vast majority of cases no single cause can be shown to be responsible for back pain and have discussed what this means for back pain prevention. You must always be suspicious of doctrinaire advice, whoever gives it. The only really sound advice is for you to do what you want to, but to stop it if it hurts!

Turning to treatments, we indicated not only that how they work is almost always unknown, but that several may be operating at once, and no one can tell precisely which. With such confusion, safety is paramount; this is the reason we gave the guides to the people who offer the various treatments and to the treatments themselves. In practical terms, your motto should be, 'Never give up!'. If one treatment fails to work for you, another may work. So you may be cautiously optimistic. But to put too much faith in any fresh approach, which may fail, could cause you unnecessary disappointment. Clinicians who are only prepared to try one treatment are almost certainly not best placed to help you.

We explained the *chronic pain state* and what it means; that, if clinicians sometimes cannot cure your pain, they can at least help you to live a normal or nearly normal life despite it. Moreover, this is done by helping you to help yourself. This means that *you* are crucial to *your* recovery, as is *your* attitude and how *you* handle *your* own situation. Finally, despair in the face of pain is not justified; as we have shown in chapter 13, the results in terms of restoring you to a normal life are really pretty good.

You may still feel that the scene is bleak; but it is now changing for the better. Everybody connected with the diagnosis and management of pain acknowledges that the present medical response is inadequate. All agree that medical training could, and must, be improved. The multi-disciplinary pain clinic is a relatively recent medical development. A few years ago, for example, the Primary Care Rheumatology Society was formed to raise standards of teaching of rheumatology in general practice. In fact, a diploma in Primary Care Rheumatology involving the Society is currently being planned. One of the five subjects will be Back Pain, which is a first at university level. Moreover, the identification by the government in 1992 of back pain as a potential key area of concern has been very helpful. As you will see, there is a wind of change blowing, and it is very much to your advantage.

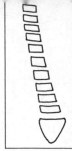

Back pain during pregnancy

Back pain felt by women early in pregnancy is often due to the womb being tilted back, and this should stop after about three months.

During pregnancy, hormones soften the ligaments to help make the pelvis mobile for birth and this may further increase the chances of back pain.

Women may also get shooting pains in their legs and buttocks because of changes in the spine. Pregnant women should reduce their chance of back pain by wearing low-heeled shoes and watching their posture; if women experience pain on lying down they should lie on their sides with their knees bent up and supported by a pillow.

A woman is vulnerable immediately after birth because the ligaments are still soft and the abdominal muscles weak. Once the baby is born women should be aware of the potential dangers to their backs from the constant bending and lifting required when looking after children. (Follow the rules on page 105). When bathing a baby or changing a nappy, kneel on the floor rather than bending from the waist.

Get as much help as you can with the household chores, and take every opportunity to rest – when your baby sleeps, you relax too!

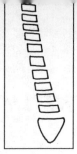

Sport and back pain

We have considered the following sporting activities:

Athletics	Jogging
Badminton	Lacrosse
Baseball	Martial arts
Boxing	Netball
Cricket	Riding
Cycling	Rowing
Dancing	Rugby football
Fencing	Skiing
Football	Squash
Fitness programmes	Swimming
Golf	Tennis
Gymnastics	Waterskiing
Hang-gliding	Windsurfing
Hockey	

You may be surprised to learn that most sports result in very little back pain when compared with the number of knee and ankle injuries. Back injuries that do occur are most often the result of collision between players in team games like rugby. In order to avoid repetition, only general advice is offered below, leaving you to interpret it for your chosen activity.

If you have back pain, or a history of previous back pain, it is important for you to warm up properly before exerting yourself in any sport. This means it is essential that you do some serious stretching and circuit training before taking to the field or track. If this hurts, *stop training at once and do not compete at all.* It may be disappointing to pull out of a game, but it is vital, if you are to avoid trouble.

Some activities, like rowing and waterskiing, are more likely than others to cause back injury. Here adequate preparation will pay off. On the other hand, no amount of preparation will protect you from hurting your back in a rugby scrum.

We feel that we should warn you about fitness clubs, as they can be breeding grounds for back pain, although they set out in part to try to prevent it. The well-run fitness club will start with a very full check on your fitness, and then work out a personal programme for you, which will depend upon what you want to achieve. You will then be taught exactly what to do. Your programme should not hurt you, and if any exercise does hurt, you must stop it at once. Remember that exercises such as sit-ups or touching your toes can be harmful. The good fitness club will have adequate supervision in the gymnasium or fitness room, so that any bad habit you may develop will be spotted early on and corrected. To summarise, the good fitness club may be a great boon to you, while the poor one may even cause you a back problem.

Safe exercises

As we said in chapter 8, exercises are the commonest therapy offered for back pain. However, exercises such as touching your toes or sit-ups can *cause* you back trouble. As always, our advice is to avoid excessive or strenuous movements and stop immediately any activity hurts. Here we give just two simple back exercises which are perfectly safe and may do you good.

LYING EXERCISE

Lie on your back, with your hands linked over your upper tummy. Keeping your knees straight, lift both legs off the floor, at the same time lifting your head and shoulders. Hold this position for about ten seconds, gently go back to your starting position and rest for five seconds. Repeat. You must do this exercise night and morning, without fail, starting with four repetitions, adding two more each week until you reach a maximum of twenty, and then continue for the rest of your life.

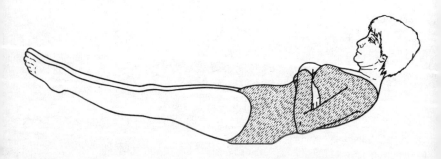

STANDING EXERCISE

Stand with your feet about eighteen inches (50cm) apart, and with your toes turned slightly inwards. Turn the palms of your hands to the front, and then twist them round, forcing your thumbs backwards, at the same time tightening the muscles of your buttocks hard. Hold this position for about ten seconds, relax for about five seconds, and repeat. As with the lying exercise, you must repeat this night and morning, starting with four

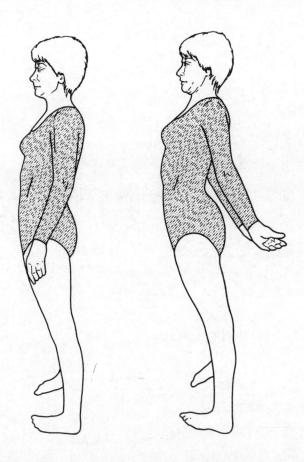

repetitions adding two each week to a maximum of twenty, and continuing them for life.

You may well find the few minutes each day spent in this way pays a worthwhile dividend.

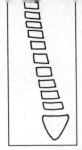

Glossary

Acute or chronic. All pain has a beginning, then runs its course and usually comes to an end. *Acute* means that the course is short, while *chronic* means that the course is long. Strictly speaking, *acute* does not mean that your pain is severe, although it is often used in this way. Both words, *acute* and *chronic* describe how long you feel your pain, rather than how much it hurts, though when pain is said to be *acute* it is often severe. If your pain begins with an injury, we talk of its onset being *sudden.* On the other hand, if it begins slowly and only later gets worse, we say its onset is *gradual.* See *chronic.*

Adjustment. This means putting something into working order. It is used in a special sense by some manipulators, i.e. *adjustment* of a joint. By this they mean that they are putting something back into its place. We do not use the term, as there is usually no proof that a particular bone is out of place to begin with!

Alexander Technique. Alexander Technique teachers use hand contact and verbal instructions to teach how to avoid preparatory tightening before movement and eliminate the harmful habits which sometimes cause back pain.

Ankylosing spondylitis. This is an important disease, not because it is common, but because its long-term effects may be serious. Its treatment is usually straightforward and should be started as soon as possible. It is used to be believed that ankylosing spondylitis was very much more likely to affect men than women, but this has been shown not to be so. Apart from pain, which may be severe if left untreated, or wrongly treated, this disease may cause long-term loss of movement and deformity. Diagnosis is not simple and it must include taking a detailed history and examination, with X-rays as well as laboratory tests. See *kyphosis*.

Annulus fibrosus. The *annulus fibrosus* is a tough, slightly elastic ring. It is an integral part of the intervertebral disc, which contains a jelly-like substance called the *nucleus pulposus*. The annulus fibrosus plays a part in spinal movements. See figure 4 on page 13.

Arthritis. *Arthritis* means inflammation of a joint, but is often wrongly used. *Arthritis* may result from injury, from infection or from particular diseases, such as rheumatoid arthritis. Many forms of arthritis get completely better, with or without treatment. But to describe as *arthritis* the wear and tear spinal changes which we all experience in middle or later life is quite wrong. The word *arthritis* may make you think of finishing in a wheelchair, but the chance of this happening is very small indeed. The word *arthritis* should only be used with an accurate label, to explain what sort of *arthritis* is meant.

Articular neurology. This is the study of the nerve supply to the joints and has recently revealed a great deal about how pain is felt and which structures the pain may be coming from.

Articular processes. These are two pairs of bony protrusions on the vertebrae. See figure 2 on page 11.

Blocked joint. Osteopaths and chiropractors find the concept of a *blocked joint* useful, although the idea is not universally accepted. When an osteopath, or other manipulator, feels a difference in movement between one vertebra and its two neighbours he or she claims to have found a blocked joint. But differences in movement between one vertebra and the next are wide, and these differences do not necessarily mean that there is anything wrong with you! There is no accepted normal range of movement. As it is the case that you cannot show what is normal, neither can you show a range of movement to be abnormal. So *blocked joint* can never be a scientifically proven diagnosis.

Bone out of place. Again, this is a concept used by osteopaths and chiropractors, although the idea is not accepted by orthodox clinicians. Bones, like noses, are never exactly the same shape in different people, and therefore a difference in knobbliness between one side and the other may be due either to a bone being out of place, or to a perfectly normal difference in shape. These differences are nearly always so small that X-rays do not show them, and they cannot therefore help in making a diagnosis.

Carpal tunnel syndrome. This condition causes pain/altered sensations in the hand. Referred back pain can produce these symptoms and give rise to misdiagnosis. See page 39.

Chronic. See *Acute or Chronic.*

Chronic pain state. This term is applied to the unhappy situation in which pain cannot be cured, despite the best endeavours of various clinicians, and may well apply to the back pain sufferer; many treatments will have been tried and failed, leading to depression and a feeling of helplessness. Never accept that there is nothing that can be done for you if you are in this group of pain sufferers; ask your clinician to refer you to a pain clinic, where you will find a variety of people highly experienced in the treatment of chronic (long-term) pain.

Coccyx. The *coccyx* is a bone which is like a rudimentary tail at the base of the spine and is made of fused vertebrae. See figure 1 on page 10.

Cognition. Psychologists use the term *cognition* to describe the way *you* understand *your* pain. Pain has different implications for different people, largely depending on their particular situation or circumstances. As a result of these differences, people react individually.

Cranial osteopathy. It is possible that the bones of your skull may move, but no one has ever proved that this happens in the adult. It is an osteopathic idea that such movements can be felt by the examiner. Further, it is claimed that, by skilled manipulation of the skull, not only these bones, but, through the attachment of tissues, the *sacrum*, the bone at the bottom of your spine, can be moved and produce important effects on blood flow and the fluid that surrounds your brain and spinal cord. While these ideas may be true, there is no scientific evidence to support them. Most doctors would think the ideas pretty far-fetched, and you would be well advised to view them with some caution. Here we come to a very important point. Because most doctors cannot accept these ideas, many of them reject osteopathy and osteopaths in general. This is unreasonable, though understandable. Many thousands of patients receive treatment from osteopaths which they find very satisfactory, for it often relieves their pain. If you have severe pain, you are first interested in getting rid of it and theories do not really matter to you. All groups of people involved in treating your back have some ideas which may be suspect, and these must be looked at critically. But you should not dismiss any group because you disagree with some of what they say. This applies to doctors, as much as to anybody else. In fact, the disc pressing on a nerve explanation is probably the worst offender – and that was a medical idea!

Crossed tendons or nerves. This is a nonsense for the same reason that 'knotted muscles' are imaginary. No such thing can possibly happen. See *Knotted muscles*.

Diagnosis. This is what is wrong with you and the tissue it comes from, i.e. the *what* and the *where* of your problem. It must be distinguished from the cause of your problem, which is *why* something went wrong.

Disc protrusion or disc lesion. These terms are often used. *Disc protrusion* means that some part of the intervertebral disc is sticking out. While this may sometimes be true, it is extremely difficult to show, for its symptoms can have several other causes. It also commonly occurs without giving you any pain at all. *Disc lesion* means that there is something wrong with an intervertebral disc. See *Slipped disc and Prolapsed disc.*

Dura mater. The *dura mater* is the protective sheath surrounding the spinal cord. See figure 7 on page 16.

Fibrositis. It has been suggested that fibrositis is an inflammation of fibrous tissue, but there is no evidence for any such thing! The term has been used for many years without proof, and it should be dropped. As far as the back sufferer is concerned, it describes a painful, tender knob in the soft tissues, such as muscle. Nonetheless, *fibrositis* is still a widely used term, both by doctors and by the public, and it has other names, which may cause more confusion. *Trigger points* is one such name. While trigger points may be important in trying to find out where something has gone wrong, they are not in themselves a diagnosis, and it is quite wrong to use the expressions *trigger points* or *fibrositis* in this way. Nevertheless, treatment of these painful points by injection with local anaesthetic and steroid is often helpful. Simply sticking a needle into them often helps, as does acupuncture.

Fracture. This word is often used wrongly. It means that a bone is broken. A *hairline fracture* is one which is very fine, possibly difficult to see on X-ray, with no displacement or separation of the two parts of the fractured bone.

A *compound fracture* is one in which a fragment of bone has pierced the skin. A *simple fracture* is one in which this has not happened. A comminuted fracture is one where a bone has split into several pieces.

Gynaecological backache. This is a vague diagnosis, suggesting that your particular backache is due to one of a number of different gynaecological problems. It can be true. It is now possible to explain how backache may be caused by problems coming from the reproductive organs and other systems of the body, such as the gut or waterworks. It may be difficult to show where the pain does come from, but no possibility must be disgarded so that mistakes in treatment may be avoided.

Hypermobility. This simply means that a joint moves more easily and has a greater range of movement than normal. This sounds pretty convincing, until you consider how you can show what is normal. Of course, you cannot do this! This we have already discussed under *blocked joint*, arguing that, if you cannot be sure what is normal, abnormal means nothing. There is, however, a condition called the *hypermobility syndrome* in which there is hyperextension of the knees and fingers and recurrent dislocation of the knee caps and shoulders. This is obviously a different ball game.

Hypomobility. This means that a joint moves less easily and has a smaller range of movement than normal. Convincing though this may sound, it is almost meaningless for the same reason that *hypermobility* and *blocked joint*, are meaningless. Some doctors and most osteopaths and chiropractors believe that to restore joint mobility to normality is the key to the relief of your pain. Once again, this theory has never been scientifically proved. Movements, such as bending forwards, backwards or to either side, may be restricted if they cause you pain, and they will be improved if the pain gets better. They may also be restricted in disease and ageing. But you still cannot show what is normal.

Intervertebral disc. The *intervertebral disc* joins two vertebral bodies together. See figure 3 on page 12.

Knotted muscles. This just does not make sense! As both ends of every muscle are firmly attached to the parts of your body they are intended to move or fix (usually to bone), knotting is obviously impossible. *Muscle tone*, or how much a muscle is contracted, varies a lot and is affected by a number of things, including both interference with its nerve supply and emotional factors. Differences in muscle tone can often be felt by the examiner, and it is probably this which gave rise to the mistaken idea that muscles may be knotted. It is no more than a rather dramatic description of what may be felt.

Kyphosis. This term describes forward bending of your spine, which may be permanent or a habit. While an upright, military bearing is not altogether a good thing, other than on the parade ground, neither is the 'droopy stoop' which is *kyphosis*. It may be due to no more than bad habit, but it may be due to underlying disease. See entries under *Ankylosing spondylitis, Osteochondritis, Osteoporosis* and *Scheuermann's disease*.

Kyphus. This is a fixed, local, forward bend of the spine. It may be the result of abnormality which has been present since childhood, or it may be the result of disease. Its cause should be looked for, as it may be treatable.

Laminae. These join the vertebral body to the articular processes.

Lateral canals. The *lateral canals* are two holes which run sideways between each pair of vertebrae. They protect the nerve roots as they branch out from the spinal cord to the rest of the body.

Ligamentous strain. The strain of a ligament is an attractive idea, but difficult to define and impossible to show. The reason is that the same pain may be produced in different parts of your body, and showing which part is extremely difficult. If it were possible to put a test strain on a particular ligament, it might then be possible to prove that ligamentous strain was true, but this is something which cannot be done. Once again, much has been written about this idea, and certain treatments rely upon it. Such treatments may work, but nobody understands why.

Ligaments. The *ligaments* are strong, fibrous and inelastic bands which hold the bones of the skeleton together and add strength to all the joints. There are seven which support the spine. See figures 6a and 6b on page 14.

Lumbago. *Lumbago* means pain in your back, between your last pair of ribs and your buttocks. It is a perfectly good word, but it says nothing at all about the cause of your pain. It is not a diagnosis, only a label saying where it hurts. Because there are many causes of lumbago, there can, of course, be no particular treatment for it.

Lumbar roll. This refers to a firm roll made of foam (or a rolled towel or rolling pin) used to maintain the *lumbar lordosis* (a natural curve of the spine). The roll is placed in the small of the back and can be very helpful to back pain sufferers.

Manipulation. Strictly speaking, this means *using the hands*. It is understood in a number of different ways by different people. It is used by manipulators to mean moving a part of your spine as a treatment for getting rid of spinal pain. *Manipulation* can be used on other joints. There are several schools of manipulation, each with its own ideas as to how manipulation should be done. The names *Cyriax*, *Maitland* and *McKenzie* are often heard in the United Kingdom. You may also have heard of osteopathic and chiropractic manipulation, and you may have heard the terms manipulation with thrust and without thrust. There is no clear proof that one method is better than another.

Mechanoceptors. The *mechanoceptors* are nerve endings which tell the brain, via the nerves to the spinal cord, *where* pain is being felt. If there are enough messages from the *mechanoceptors*, the pain messages from the *nociceptors* will not get through to the brain and no pain will be felt. This may explain why people suffering from a serious injury may not experience pain until some time after the injury occurred – the messages telling *where* the injury was inflicted will not let the pain messages through to the brain.

Mobile segment. The *mobile segment* is the term given to two adjacent vertebrae and all that joins and separates them. All the structures in a mobile segment have to move at the same time. See figure 10 on page 19.

Mobilisation. This means increasing movement. It has been brought into the osteopathic and chiropractic vocabulary as meaning a gentle form of manipulation of joints. Others have also adopted this usage. We use it only in its original sense.

Musculoskeletal medicine. See *Orthopaedic medicine*.

Neurology. The term *neurology* is the name given to the study of nerves. The neurology of pain is very complicated but recent research has yielded a large amount of information which is now used in pain prevention and relief.

Nociceptors. These are the nerve endings which, when stimulated, either chemically or mechanically, send pain messages to the brain. If the messages from the *mechanoceptors* (messages which tell *where* something is happening in the body) are stronger than the nociceptors, pain is not felt. This process is the basis of many pain relief techniques.

Nucleus pulposus. This is the jelly-like substance contained in the *annulus fibrosus*. See figure 4 on page 13.

Orthopaedic medicine. This is the branch of medicine which deals with the problems of your bones, joints and related parts, without the use of surgery. It is sometimes called *locomotor medicine* or, better, *musculoskeletal medicine*.

Osteoarthritis. This is not a good word. *Osteo-* suggests that it is primarily to do with bones, *arthr-* suggests that it is to do with a joint, while *-itis* means that it is an inflammation. In fact, although it does describe something to do with a joint, the chief process is one of wear and tear and not of inflammation, and it is only late in the day that the bone is affected. The part inflammation plays in this condition is still not fully understood. *See arthritis and osteoarthrosis.*

Osteoarthrosis. This is a better word than *osteoarthritis* because, although it suggests that it is mainly bone that is affected, *osteo-*, it is certainly to do with a joint, *arthr-* and *-osis* implies that there is something wrong. This is the wear and tear which is a part of growing older, and it does not usually mean either pain or disability.

Osteochondritis. In man, the cause of this disease is unknown, but it leads to an inflammation of part of a joint and results in pain and deformity. The *chondr-* part means that it is the cartilage which is mainly affected.

Osteopathic lesion. This word is supposed to describe what is wrong with the way a joint works, usually that it is hypomobile, though hypomobility cannot be proved. The osteopathic lesion describes what *may* happen, and tries to explain what is at present unknown. We prefer to use the expression *painful segmental disorder*, because it says no more and no less than what we *do* know; *painful* because you say so, a *disorder* because pain, whatever its cause, is a disorder; *segmental* because we believe that the spinal level or levels at which your trouble arises can usually be found and treated.

Osteophytes. These are bony outgrowths which appear at the edges of ageing joints. They develop over a long time, as part of the process of growing old. They can be seen on X-ray, but are usually of little importance, as they usually cause no trouble at all. However, they can cause considerable pain, if their size and position interferes with other parts, for example with nerves.

Osteoporosis. This means a weakening of bone by reduction of the amount of calcium it contains. The more calcium you have in your bones, the denser they appear on X-ray, and the stronger they are likely to be. If you have *osteoporosis* it means that your bones are less dense than they should be. This becomes more common as you get older and is more common in women. The osteoporotic bone is weak and may be damaged under ordinary stresses, so if *osteoporosis* is suspected any treatment must be gentle and the cause must be sought and found.

Painful segmental disorder. This is the term we use for the pain you most commonly have in your back. *You* know it is painful, *we* usually have a pretty good idea which segmental level it comes from, and, if it hurts, it must be out of order! It makes no claim to be a diagnosis, but it is of practical use to the doctor in deciding what treatment to suggest.

Pathology. This is the study of how things go wrong in your body. See *Physiology.*

Pectoral girdle. This is made up of the collar bone and shoulder blades, together with their attachments to the spine. See figure 8a on page 17.

Pedicles. These are bony outgrowths which jut out from the vertebral body. See figure 2 on page 11.

Pelvic girdle. This is at the base of the spine and is made up of the pubic bones and the illiac bones. See figure 8b on page 17.

(Physical) sign. This is any abnormality we find when we examine your back. It is different from a symptom, which is something *you feel.* Finding physical signs helps us to understand your case and to decide where your pain is coming from.

Physiology. This is the study of how your body normally works. See *Pathology.*

Placebo effect. This occurs when you get relief from a treatment which has no apparent medical properties because you *believe* the treatment will relieve your pain or symptoms.

Posterior vertebral joints. These are pairs of small joints. See figure 3 on page 12.

Prolapsed (intervertebral) disc. This term is used when the *annulus fibrosus* is so badly damaged that some of the *nucleus pulposus* is squeezed through the outer layers of the disc into the spinal canal. Here it may interfere with the nervous system, sometimes pressing on the spinal cord or on one or more of the nerve roots coming from it. Unfortunately, tests for this condition are not always very helpful, and this makes diagnosis difficult. A disc bulging, though not strictly prolapsed, may cause pain, while a true prolapse may cause you no trouble at all! Some authorities describe protrusions as *hard* or *soft*, and claim to be able to tell the difference between them. No evidence has been put forward to support this idea. The prolapsed disc certainly does exist, but it is rarely possible to prove it, except during an operation.

Putting a bone or disc back. We have said how difficult it is to show that a bone or disc is out of place. Putting it back must be just as difficult to prove. Because of this problem, we do not use this expression.

Referred pain. This means pain felt in a place it does not come from. For example, you may feel pain in your arm which really comes from your neck, or pain down your leg which comes from your back.

Referred tenderness. *Tenderness* is pain caused by pressure which normally would not hurt. *Referred tenderness* means that this pain is produced as a result of a disorder elsewhere, in exactly the same way as referred pain is felt at a distance from where it arises. Referred tenderness may help us to find the spinal level at which your pain arises.

Rheumatism. It is impossible to define rheumatism precisely, because it covers a large group of different diseases. What these diseases have in common is that they involve bones, joints and muscles. If we wish to refer to one particular disease, such as *rheumatoid arthritis*, we give it a proper label. Otherwise we do not use the term.

Rheumatoid arthritis. *Rheumatoid arthritis* is a particular disease which, untreated, runs a variable course, and which is not fully understood. Diagnosis is by clinical examination, X-rays and laboratory tests. It is an important disease for two reasons: first because it is common and may become severely disabling, and second because, if you have it, your neck *must not* be manipulated, as this could prove very dangerous indeed. If you have this condition, you will probably find yourself under the care of a rheumatologist.

Rhizolysis. This is a treatment which has been used for many years. Its object is to remove the nervous pathway conducting your pain, in particular in chronic pain coming from the small posterior joints of the spine. It is performed by almost literally 'frying' the nerves. It usually produces good results, although they cannot be guaranteed.

Rhizotomy. This has the same aim as rhizolysis. It is performed by cutting the nerves with a specially designed knife. Results of these two treatments vary because there is an overlap of the nerve supply of the posterior joints. So that cutting or 'frying' one or two nerves may not achieve any improvement at all, for other nerves may be doing the job. Like rhizolysis, the result is usually good, but it cannot be guaranteed.

Sacral hiatus. This is a hole at the bottom of the sacrum. Caudal epidural injections are administered via this.

Sacrum. The *sacrum* is a triangular bone at the back of the pelvis made up of five fused vertebrae. See figure 1 on page 10.

Scheuermann's disease. This disease causes the spine to bend; its cause is unknown, and how bad it is is very variable. Most cases are very mild and are often not noticed when they begin. It is common for it to be diagnosed many years later, on routine X-ray, when the typical damage to the vertebral body is seen. The relatively rare, severe cases need urgent treatment by splinting the spine to prevent deformity. Because the deformity is a forward bending of your spine, the splint is designed to keep your back straight until the active phase of the disease is over. If you have this disease, you should never be manipulated in the active stage, as this may delay the correct treatment.

Sciatica. This means pain down the back of your leg, maybe as far as the foot. This is in the area supplied by the *greater sciatic nerve*, which is how it gets its name. Like lumbago, it is no more than a statement of where your pain is felt. It says nothing about the cause of the problem, and usually has little to do with the sciatic nerve.

Sclerosant therapy. This treatment is intended to toughen up ligaments in your back thought to be lax. Because there is no proof of this, and as it is very painful, it is less commonly used nowadays than it used to be.

Scoliosis. This is the word applied to the deformity of your spine in which there is a combination of sidebending and twisting. It may be present at birth or develop later. It may be slight or quite marked. In some cases it may be combined with a tilt of your pelvis. In others it may be due to a difference in leg length. Its cause is usually unknown and in mild cases, you will live with it in the happy ignorance that you have anything wrong!

Slipped disc. This term causes much confusion. The importance of the disc as a cause of back pain was first suggested in 1932, when an American surgeon found that what he had cut out at operation was part of an intervertebral disc. He jumped to the conclusion that this must be the cause of lumbago and sciatica, a theory immediately taken up by the medical profession, although never proved to be a common cause of these problems. In the following forty years over three thousand professional papers were published on the subject, but none has provided satisfactory evidence that the disc is a common cause of back pain. Indeed, recent work shows that the disc is at fault in no more than one case in twenty of lumbago and sciatica! This is an interesting example of a 'diagnostic fashion' for which the orthodox medical profession is largely to blame. A generation ago it was *the* medical back pain diagnosis. Now, happily, it is less often made by informed doctors. The disc is really a sort of semi-hydraulic shock-absorber, and it does not slip, pop in and out, or perform any of the rather odd things said about it. It does change with age, becoming less effective as a shock-absorber, and it may be damaged in a number of ways, including by some exercises and treatments. But there remains no evidence that we put it back, any more than there was evidence that it was out. It never slips!

Soft tissue techniques. This is the modern word for 'handling' treatments which do not involve or include manipulation. Well known to all physiotherapists, these techniques include various forms of massage.

Spinal canal. This is the hole down the middle of the vertebrae. The spinal canal contains and protects the spinal cord.

Spinal cord. This is made up of nerve material and is an extension of the brain. It conveys information to the brain from all parts of the body. See figure 7 on page 16.

Spinal level. This is the level of each vertebra. Local physical examination can reveal an abnormal spinal level and indicate an appropriate treatment.

Spinal stenosis. This means narrowing of the spinal canal, which may be important, for it leaves less room for the soft parts, which may be squashed inside. If the degree of stenosis is great, surgical decompression may be the only effective treatment. This means cutting away whatever is squashing the soft parts.

Spinous processes. These are protrusions at the back of the vertebrae. See figure 2 on page 11.

Spondylolisthesis. This means that one vertebra has slipped forwards on the one immediately below. It is only serious if there is damage to other parts of the vertebra. If it is severe, it needs surgery *(spinal fusion)* to prevent further slip, which could damage the spinal cord. Most people with this condition remain without pain.

Spondylolysis. This is damage of any sort to that part of the vertebra which is essential for holding the package together. This is called the *pedicle*, which is the bridge between the weight-bearing joint at the front and the pair of posterior joints at each level. If this part is defective, then *spondylolisthesis* is possible. You might think of this as a slipped vertebra, rather than a slipped disc.

Spondylosis. This means the basic wear and tear changes of the vertebrae which are part of the process of growing old. Many people confuse this with spondylitis and worry about it without cause. (See *ankylosing spondylitis.*) *Spondylosis* may be seen on X-ray from the age of thirty onwards and usually has little or nothing to do with any pain you may have.

Subject report. This term is applied to your description of your pain and symptoms to a doctor or clinician. As it relies on your own experience and interpretation of your situation it can be unreliable and confuse diagnosis.

Subluxation. This means that, in a joint, one part has slipped slightly on another. It is a minor form of dislocation. Commonly used by osteopaths and chiropractors, it has rarely been proved as a cause of back pain.

Symptom. This is something you feel to be wrong with you. Pain is a *symptom*, wherever you feel it, as are stiffness, numbness and pins and needles. Symptoms always have a place – for example, you may have pain in your back or in one elbow. Description of pain is naturally very individual, and for this reason it is not very useful in our search for its cause.

Traction. This is a very old form of treatment for your spine. It involves stretching the whole or a part of it. The pull may be by hand or by some form of apparatus, sometimes using the force of gravity. It may be used for relatively short periods or, under lesser loads, for days on end. In spite of a number of ideas being put forward to explain how it works, such as sucking back a protruding nucleus into its proper place, no one has been able to prove such ideas, and we are left with insufficient knowledge to explain its successes. It helps in an unpredictable proportion of cases and it is safe. You may feel that it is currently rather unfairly neglected. A number of machines have been designed, to provide traction, including very sophisticated ones, which can be programmed to apply differing pulls at different times. There is no reason to think a traction machine which turns you upside down is doing you any more good than one that leaves you the right way up.

Transcutaneous nerve stimulation (TENS). A machine is used to deliver electrical stimulation to the mechanoceptor nerve fibres, thus blocking the perception of pain. See page 52.

Transverse processes. These are pairs of bony protrusions from the sides of the vertebrae. See figure 2 on page 11.

Trauma. This means *injury.*

Trigger points. These have been dealt with under *fibrositis.*

Vertebrae. These are the 24 bones between your skull and pelvis.

Vertebral arteries. These are the two arteries in the spine which supply blood to the brain. If you suffer from arterial disease, treatment for back pain must not involve manipulation of the neck, for fear of cutting off the blood supply to your brain.

Vertebral bodies. These are the main weight-bearing parts of your spine. See figure 10 on page 19.

Zygoapophyseal joint. This is another term for the *posterior vertebral* joints. See figure 3 on page 12.

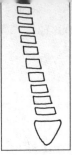

Organisations which may help

We are indebted to Dr Bryn-Jones for writing the following section on the *National Back Pain Association*.

The National Back Pain Association is the only charity solely devoted to back pain. Compared with the size of the back pain problem it is a small charity, employing the equivalent of eight staff, with a turnover of about £300,000. Founded 25 years ago by industrialist Stanley Grundy, it has three main objectives:

- To fund patient oriented scientific research into the causes and treatment of back pain.
- To educate people to use their bodies sensibly and thus reduce the incidence of pain.
- To help form and support branches through which back pain sufferers and those who care for them may receive advice and mutual help.

RESEARCH
When the Association began, it concentrated on funding back pain research. The need to include education in its objectives was realised at an early stage and the benefit of self-help recognised by the end of the 1970s. The Association now tries to devote its energies fairly evenly between its objectives, although from year to year this may vary according to the priorities at the time.

Back Pain research is not well funded in the United Kingdom. The NBPA is currently funding about £100,000 of medical research. This sum is minute compared with the amounts spent by larger charities, but because back pain is not life-threatening or emotive it is unable to attract the funds raised by more popular causes.

The NBPA is able to support research opportunities which fall outside the scope of traditional funders and even small amounts of money devoted to the right project can make all the difference. The NBPA research policy reflects the value of being multidisciplinary and the Association funds research into complementary as well as orthodox medicine, with the emphasis being on the benefit to the patient.

EDUCATION

The educational work of the NBPA is very wide. First of all it teaches those who have back pain how to help themselves. It gives them an insight into what causes back pain and how to lessen the chances of its recurring. Through our magazine, books, videos and leaflets we encourage back pain sufferers to take on the responsibility for looking after their backs, for we know that the feeling of control they gain will enhance their quality of life.

The back pain sufferer looks to us for advice in ever increasing numbers. This is especially true of the new back pain sufferer to whom back pain is a very frightening experience. We provide information about diagnosing back pain, the kinds of treatment that are available and how exercise will help. We also tell people which chairs, back supports, therapy aids and other back products are on the market and where they can get them.

Unfortunately many of the people who contact us are chronic back pain sufferers, for whom the pain is unrelenting. For most, information is no longer enough, for they have, more often than not, tried all that traditional and complementary has to offer. Sometimes we have to tell them about the work of pain clinics, but most of all we give them understanding and encouragement. Knowing that they are not alone and talking through problems puts their pain into perspective.

Secondly the National Back Pain Association teaches prevention. How to avoid getting back in the first place. How to reduce the chances of back pain happening again. We publish good ergonomic advice for all those concerned with manual handling and produce the standard text, in collaboration with the Royal College of Nursing, on handling patients. At a more popular level, the Association produces a range of leaflets extolling the virtues of back care. It starts where all good prevention programmes should, with school children and covers a range of domestic and working situations. Simple, commonsense advice to make people aware of the dangers of their backs.

SELF-HELP

The National Back Pain Association set up its first Branch in 1978. The Association recognised that back pain sufferers needed help locally. It decided to bring back pain sufferers together to share common problems and help them to gain more control over their own health. Since 1978, the Branch network has grown modestly. There are now about 30 and a similar number of Local Contacts.

The NBPA Branches provide a great deal of practical help. Through their meetings they explain the nature of back pain and what therapies can do to help. They sustain back pain sufferers and their carers and many provide exercise and hydrotherapy classes. And, of course, through their fundraising for back pain research, they provide the hope that one day an answer will be found.

The Branches and Membership of the National Back Pain Association also provide a necessary lobbying function. The fact that the Government is now discussing back pain is in part due to their vociferousness. When the original Health of the Nation excluded back pain from its proposals, NBPA members protested vigorously and with considerable success that it should be included in the White Paper. The back pain sufferer has strong views about back pain and the National Back Pain Association is the mouthpiece through which those views can be voiced. As a Branch Member recently wrote; 'Get in touch with a self-help group. You can do yourself more good learning how to help yourself than seeing all the GPs and specialists in the world – they don't know enough about back pain.'

JOIN THE NBPA

The National Back Pain Association urgently needs your help. Become a member and we will send you a copy of our very readable magazine TalkBack four times a year. This will keep you up to date on back pain issues and progress on research. You will also get a copy of our Annual Report and be able to vote at the AGM. In this way you can participate in decisions about how to fight back pain. But above all, you will be part of an organisation working solely for back pain sufferers and their carers; funding research, teaching back care and encouraging self-help.

For more information, write to *National Back Pain Association, 31–33 Park Road, Teddington, Middlesex TW11 0AB. Telephone: 081 977 5474.*

The *British Acupuncture Association*, 34 Alderney Street, London SW1 V4EU. Telephone: 071 834 1012, publishes a list of practitioners and a question and answer booklet on acupuncture, available from the above address at a cost of £2.30.

The *British Association of Psychotherapists*, 37 Mapesbury Road, London NW2 4HJ. Telephone: 081 452 9823, fax: 081 452 5182, will give information and advice if you are considering psychotherapy. Contact their Clinical Service at the address above.

The *British Chiropractic Association*, 29 Whitley Street, Reading, Berks RG2 0EG. Telephone: 0734 757557. All members have completed a full-time four-year course which gives a BSc degree in Chiropractic, followed by one year's work under the supervision of a trained chiropractor.

The *British Homoeopathic Association*, 27a Devonshire Street, London W1N 1RJ. Telephone: 071 935 2163, will supply a register of doctors with varying levels of homoeopoathic training.

The *British League Against Rheumatism* (BLAR), is an umbrella organisation, representing the interests of all those connected with rheumatology. It is a member of the **European League Against Rheumatism** (EULAR). It is also affiliated to the **International League Against Rheumatism** (ILAR). BLAR has two main sections: the scientific section, consisting very largely of rheumatologists, and a community section, made up of organisations like **Arthritis Care**, the **Scoliosis Association**, the **National Ankylosing Spondylitis Society**, etc. These organisations are made up of sufferers from the particular conditions their titles suggest. BLAR operates from 3 St Andrew's Place, Regents Park, London NW1 4LB. Telephone: 071 224 3739.

It is both interesting and encouraging that **Arthritis Care** (for example), is now growing in membership at a rate of something like 150 per week. It has its headquarters at 18 Stephenson Way, London NW1 2HD. Telephone: 071 916 1500. An information/counselling service is available on the main telephone number 10.00 AM–4.00 PM on weekdays, and a FREEPHONE helpline is available on 0800 289170 from 12.00–4.00 PM.

The **Scoliosis Association** is to be found at 2 Ivebury Court, 323–327 Latimer Road, London W10 6RA. Telephone: 081 964 5343.

The **National Ankylosing Spondylitis Society** is at 5 Grosvenor Crescent, London SW1X 7ER. Telephone: 071 235 9585.

The *British Medical Association (BMA)*, BMA House, Tavistock Square, London WC1H 9JP. Telephone: 071 387 4499. BMA is a trade union for doctors and does not give advice to patients or the general public, but has a public information service.

The *Chartered Society of Physiotherapy*, 14 Bedford Row, London WC1R 4ED. Telephone: 071 242 1941. Training is a three-year full-time course (most now being degree courses) leading to qualification as a Chartered Physiotherapist.

The *Council for Complementary and Alternative Medicine* (CCAM), 179 Gloucester Place, London NW1 6DX. Telephone: 071 724 9103, will send information on recognised practitioners on receipt of a stamped addressed envelope and a cheque or postal order for £1.00.

The *Institute of Musculo-skeletal Medicine*, Medical Centre, Hythe, Southampton, Hants SO4 5ZB. Please address all letters to the Secretary.

The *National Institute of Medical Herbalists*, 9 Palace Gate, Exeter EX1 1JA. Telephone: 0392 213899, will send a list of registered medical herbalists, an application to the Secretary at the address above.

The *Natural Medicine Society*, which can provide advice about all kinds of alternative approaches to back pain, can be contacted at Edith Lewis House, Ilkeston, Derbyshire DE7 8EJ. Telephone: 0602 329454.

The Osteopathic Information Service, 37 Soho Square, London W1V 5DG. Telephone 071 439 7177, has factsheets which explain what osteopathy is and how to find an osteopath and give further general information about osteopathy and the conditions it can treat.

The *Society of Homoeopaths*, 2 Artizan Road, Northampton NN1 4HU. Telephone: 0604 21400, will supply a register of professional practitioners.

The *Society of Teachers of the Alexander Technique* (STAT), 20 London House, 266 Fulham Road, London SW10 9EL. Telephone: 071 351 0828, has a list of qualified teachers. Clients are taught how to improve their posture and everyday movements to eliminate harmful habits which are sometimes the cause of pain.

Suppliers of back pain products

Anatomia Ltd, 21 Hampstead Road, London NW1 33A. Telephone: 071 387 5700, Fax: 071 387 3916, has a showroom and produces a mail order catalogue.

The Back Shop, 24 New Cavendish Street, London W4M 7LH. Telephone: 071 935 9120, offers a free 'posture assessment' and a mail order catalogue.